FUTUREPROOF

Also by Davinia Taylor

It's Not a Diet
Hack Your Hormones

FUTUREPROOF

BUILD RESILIENCE, FEEL YOUNGER, LIVE LONGER

DAVINIA TAYLOR

First published in Great Britain in 2025 by Orion Spring,
an imprint of The Orion Publishing Group Ltd
Carmelite House, 50 Victoria Embankment
London EC4Y 0DZ

An Hachette UK Company

The authorised representative in the EEA is Hachette Ireland,
8 Castlecourt Centre, Dublin 15, D15 XTP3, Ireland (email: info@hbgi.ie)

5 7 9 10 8 6

Reviewed for scientific accuracy by Dr Tamsin Lewis @sportiedoc wellgevity.com

A CIP catalogue record for this book is
available from the British Library.

ISBN (Export Trade Paperback) 978 1 3987 0965 2
ISBN (Ebook) 978 1 3987 0966 9
ISBN (Audio) 978 1 3987 0967 6

Typeset by Input Data Services Ltd, Bridgwater, Somerset

Printed in Great Britain by Clays Ltd, Elcograf S.p.A.

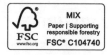

MIX
Paper | Supporting
responsible forestry
FSC® C104740

www.orionbooks.co.uk

CONTENTS

Dedicated to my lovely mum, and my mother-in-law.
Taken too soon – we miss you every day.

INTRODUCTION

HOW OLD ARE YOU REALLY?

Recently, I found out that my body is twenty years old. I'm not kidding! Obviously, I know I'm in my forties, I'm not a lunatic. I've got the kids, the divorce and the experience to show for it. But when I took a blood test from GlycanAge – a company who are able to test the chronic inflammation in our cells at a molecular level – my *biological age* came back as twenty (not to be confused with chronological age, which would tell you I am forty-seven). I was like, *WTF, seriously?* Of course, I was pleased, but it really floored me, especially considering how old I used to feel.

Feeling older when I was younger

I'll explain the difference between chronological vs biological age. Chronological age is how many years old we actually are; how many years we've been wandering around this planet, annoying people and compulsively spending money on useless clutter (which I'm now hoarding)! Biological age is how old our cells are, based on the levels of inflammation and damage they have.[1] Sometimes the two match up, but sometimes they can be really, really, different. You know how you could meet an eighty-year-old woman, but she's got the energy and life of a forty-year-old? Or come across somebody in their twenties but who looks and behaves so much older? Almost flatline in enthusiasm? To be honest, that was me when I was thirty-five. I felt absolutely *awful*.

Although I was five years sober by then, if you've read my previous books, you'll know that I replaced alcohol with a sugar and carbohydrate addiction – and, naturally, some shopping! The consequences of that aged me not only physically, but mentally and emotionally. Forget running, I could barely push my toddler around in the pram without a lot of huffing and puffing. Everything was arduous and mundane. I felt hopeless, brain-foggy, with no optimism or get up and go – even emptying the dishwasher felt like too much. (And to be fair, I still hate that task, which seems to have been allocated to me alone for some reason!) My joints were achy, swollen and spongy, and I was constantly exhausted.

Feeling like this – old before my time, weak, moody – became my norm. I didn't realise that I was overfed yet undernourished, and chronically inflamed. (I'll explain inflammation in more detail as we go on, but for now, it meant having less energy and more detrimental body fat. Yes, there are different types of body fat! More on that later, too.) I can guarantee that if I'd taken a biological age test *then*, I would have come out as at least twenty years older than I really was – *at least* late fifties.

Since then, as many of you probably already know, I've completely changed my approach to my health, drawing instead on real scientific research and seeing what works for me rather than the one-size-fits-all received wisdom. I look for the latest data with an eye on our ancestral evolution. I feel better now, in my late forties, than I ever did in my teens, twenties or thirties. So I took this test because it really drills down on what we're going to be exploring in this book – **how to age well, and live a long, healthy, vibrant life.**

Why we fear ageing

Let's be honest – right now, we've got a pretty negative approach to getting older in our society. We dread it. We are conditioned to believe that ageing is going to be horrible, with no positives, and subsequently we have all these negative connotations attached to it. Getting older in our minds equals being weak, unattractive, suffering with ill health, discomfort and pain. This is so traumatising to us, we actually ignore it. We're in complete denial that we're going to get older, so we don't prepare for the inevitable and help ourselves mitigate the risks.

And the scary thing is, we're not wrong to think like this! Data shows us that although we're living longer overall, we're spending more of our lives sick. In England and Wales, women spend 23 per cent of their lives – which averages out at close to twenty years – in poor health.[2] I mean, what the fuck? Genuine question: what's the point in all of us living till ninety, or a hundred, if a huge number of those final two decades are full of misery?

The weird thing is, we humans are pretty ambivalent and passive about this. We've been conditioned by society, culture, by modern medicine, to think that this is inevitable. That there's no way around it – we'll either end up having cancer, dementia, or myriad disabilities and have gone through fifteen years of agony by the time we get to the end. To be honest with you, I'd much rather be in a box than have that be the end of my life. And I've seen first-hand how awful it can be, with both my mum and my mother-in-law suffering before they died. We all think it's sad, but *Oh well, that's just the way it is*. But it's not. It doesn't have to be.

Healthspan, not lifespan

It *is* possible to live a long, healthy life where we're full of energy, dynamism and enjoying ourselves right up to the end. That's true longevity. And the big focus now in innovative medicine is about increasing *healthspan* rather than just our lifespan. Healthspan is simply the number of years we live in good health, able to do what we want free of chronic disease or pain. And as we've seen from the stats above (never mind our own personal and family experiences) this isn't what's happening right now.

So, how about it? What if we could live way past eighty still kicking ass, or to ninety still going on the golf course? (Or in my case, doing TK Maxx raids!) Or still swimming, or still laughing our heads off with our mates, or still going on a cruise with our partner? Whatever would look like an enjoyable and carefree life for *you*. For me, it would likely involve a lot of swearing at young people. I want to be a don't-give-a-shit old lady who is naughty AF and full of mischief and curiosity! I want to learn new things, socialise and be busy with my million grandchildren, not wither away in a chair in a nursing home, lonely and, worst of all, frightened. I want to ski with them, have fun with them, take them on a track and run with them. That's what I want to do! Why not?

We're told so often that this is *impossible*. That pain and weakness are part and parcel of getting older. In fact, it's not – and there is so much exciting research, with actionable protocols out there that show us otherwise. That's what's on my radar right now – it's a huge, exciting, busy field with incredible research coming out. This book is going to bring together the latest advice so that all of us can put ourselves in the best place to live a healthy, long life.

Why it's not about being plastic fantastic

Being youthful is about way more than aesthetics – just simply looking good. Look, I'm the last person on earth to judge someone for wanting to look their best. I completely understand and relate to the confidence boost you have when you look your best – when your hair is great, your eyes are white, your skin is clear and glowing. Of course that makes us feel good! So, I will look into what causes skin ageing, and what we can do that *isn't* just shoving filler into our cheeks at the age of thirty-nine because we've been told to avoid 'runner's face', and end up with a dent from having it dissolved a few years later (yep, *hello* – I'll tell you about that later).

We will look at what can help you look your best too, but it's not about looking plastic fantastic. When I meet somebody, I don't just think about their appearance as a measure of how youthful they are. It's about the chat, it's about how engaged and positive they are, how open to new experiences. That's what I find youthful – it's an attitude. Combined with a few years of experience, you end up with an amazing, inspiring wisdom which I really dig – and to be honest, I find way more convincing than listening to a twenty-one-year-old wannabe on TikTok, who I can't help but feel sorry for because they haven't really been challenged by life yet. Great that you're optimistic and full of beans; however, come back to me when you've gone through redundancy, divorce, kids, deaths in the family – that is when life's got real!

So, rather than be frightened of what's coming down the road, and avoiding any thoughts about it by sticking our head in the sand and reaching for that Twix, we're going to take a proactive approach to our future. We're going to flip the received wisdom about ageing on its head. Instead, we'll explore what scientific research shows will extend our healthspan, not just our lifespan. We all want to make the years we have on this earth fabulous. None of us *want* to have a crap last decade of our lives and then die in pain, do we? So, maximising our healthspan is paramount.

Reality check – it's not about living for ever

Right, I'm just going to make it 100 per cent clear before we move on any further – this book isn't going to be about stopping time or 'cheating' death in some way. That's not what longevity is about, some deluded billionaire tech bro trying to spend his way into living for ever. Not at all. Of course we can't escape death! The only certainty in this life is that we're all going to frigging die.

But what we can do is *slow down* the hallmarks of ageing and steady our health decline. We can help lay the foundations for a healthy old age so that we don't end up living our final years in sickness and pain. And if you think *That's all very well, but I could get hit by a bus tomorrow*, then remember you're statistically much more likely to get cancer than get knocked over. And I promise you, neither you nor I want to go through what my mum went through and be dead at sixty.

I know I'm far from alone in seeing my loved ones experience a terrible death. So many of us have gone through this or are going through this right now. No wonder so many of us dread getting older – we're not frightened of death, but of 'losing our humanity', as Dr David Sinclair, a professor of genetics at Harvard, puts it. But we can change this; extend our healthspan and have an enjoyable, vital life all the way through.

Reframing ageing – is it a disease?

One of the first things I want to do with this book is reframe how we think about ageing. Like I've said, we all have so many negative connotations we associate with the process of getting older. But there's a huge amount of work – and debates – going on in medical fields right now, with increasing numbers of incredible experts and thinkers arguing that ageing is a disease.

This might sound nuts, but hang on for a mo! What we believe to be the symptoms of ageing is actually a process of disease. Ageing is behind our physical decline which impacts our quality of life. What's more, it has a specific *pathology*, which means that scientists can identify what causes it – things like stem-cell exhaustion, epigenetic alteration and telomere shortening. (Do not fret – we don't need to know all these terms, just that they are identifiable, and they are behind ageing.)

What's more, in all the big diseases like cancer and dementia, we see that ageing is a huge risk factor. In 2010 a game-changing meeting took place, where nineteen of the world's leading scientists agreed that we were entering a 'new science of ageing'. This isn't tin-hat conspiracy nonsense, this is real, peer-reviewed stuff. If you believe the idea that ageing is a disease is in the same bracket as a flat-earther conspiracy theorist, you're wrong. This is critical thinking where science is asking new questions, and so many ideas that were dismissed only a few years ago as bonkers are now scientific theory.

Defining disease – and why it's inconsistent

For example, so many things have made me reconsider how we define a 'disease'. Something I watched recently really got me thinking. It pointed out how the medical establishment classifies diseases is not consistent. In fact, it's really erratic.

For example, when it comes to types of addiction, alcohol addiction is classified as a disease,[3] but nicotine addiction *isn't*. Now that really made me sit up and go 'wow'. For me, as a recovering alcoholic? That blew my mind. I regularly sit in twelve-step meetings, and although I don't smoke, everyone else is constantly popping out for a cigarette. They've replaced one addiction with another. I asked my group what they thought about classifying one addiction as a disease but not the other, and the overall response was that this was bloody crazy! And they'd never even considered it from this perspective. This is from people who understand first-hand what these addictions are like.

And what about obesity? Since 2013, that's been classified as a disease in the US and the EU, as well as by the World Health Organization, but *not* in the UK! But this really shows us how uneven it is – not all medical practitioners agree, and *do not treat diseases exactly the same way*. If something is classified as a disease, there will then be more research and investment focused on looking at and understanding it, so if ageing does end up being defined differently, I think that's fabulous.

If you still need convincing, let's note that ideas of what a disease is have already moved on radically. Masturbation used to be considered a disease, as was homosexuality! (By the way, cornflakes were invented by Mr Kellogg to cure the 'masturbation problem' – I kid you not.) That seems insane to us now, but remember, that's 'just how it was' in the not-so-long-ago past. Life-threatening illnesses change, too. Half of Americans used to die from pneumonia, tuberculosis, flu and gastric disease. That's 'just how it was' back in 1900. But not now.

The important thing is to recognise that times change. Medicine changes. Knowledge changes. So, we need to change with it! We don't have to accept this idea that what modern medicine, i.e. our GP, tells us to do is the only 'right' way to approach longevity and treating disease.

The problems with modern medicine

These days, we're most likely to die from cancer, dementia, Alzheimer's, diabetes or cardiovascular (heart) disease. But the way we treat these diseases is bizarrely reductionist. Most modern Western medicine focuses on treating each disease separately: cutting them out, poisoning them with chemo, or blitzing them with drugs. You can easily end up suffering extra mental distress as you wait for all the dots to be joined together, and sometimes diagnoses can be missed because of how separately everything works. For example, oncologists treat cancer, endocrinologists manage diabetes, and neurologists handle dementia-related conditions. However, the interplay between these diseases and their shared underlying causes – such as inflammation, metabolic dysfunction and lifestyle factors – can be overlooked. Our medical culture was originally built on the concept of treating individual diseases, so no wonder things are segregated. But we've now got a situation where the diabetes doctors work separately from the cancer team, who work separately from the neurologists, and so on.

Loads of doctors, such as Dr Mark Hyman, are speaking out about the limitations of this system and the fact that the uncertainty that exists in the science behind these treatments can leave decision makers feeling like they're taking an 'educated guess'. Modern medicine is not infallible. If it was, 86,000 cancer patients wouldn't be misdiagnosed each year in the US, and maybe my mum and Matthew's mum would still be alive. As it is, my kids are growing up without their grandmothers. They were both vital women with tons of life and love to offer and cancer has taken both of them, one at sixty and one at seventy.

My mum's cancer misdiagnosis

I'm still so angry that my mum was misdiagnosed. They told her she had lung cancer based on the location of the tumour, without actually testing the tumour itself. She'd already had breast cancer before, when she was twenty-seven, so we were always worried it would come back. That first time, back in the late 1970s, she'd been successfully treated at a hospital in Manchester – and thank God, because I would have grown up without a mum. (My mum was a really calm, levelling presence in our family, forever mopping up my emotional outbursts.) When she got ill again, I argued with the oncologist that it was the breast cancer come back, but they insisted, 'No, it's lung cancer', and they treated her on that basis.

It made no difference. The tumour got bigger and bigger, and spread into her spine. My poor mum was in permanent agony. I was desperate to do anything I could to help her. I was prepared to sell everything I had just to keep my mum alive so she could meet her grandchild, as I was pregnant with my third son. Very firmly, I was told there was nothing else that they could do, and she was already in the best place possible.

It was just by chance that I discovered there were other options. I was living in London back then, and one day I was crying in the communal gardens when I bumped into my Iranian neighbour. She asked what was wrong, and when I told her, she said, 'Well, you have to take her to Germany!' The hospitals there were using an innovative form of personalised cancer treatment using DNA sequencing. My mum was very reluctant to go and felt loyal to the hospital at home. After all, they'd saved her life once before, and she was terrified. After twelve months of 'shooting in the dark' chemotherapy, we were told there was nothing left to try and that my mum should go home and be comfortable. Giving up wasn't an option, so we booked her into the German clinic and got her on a plane.

In Germany, the treatment was so different from the UK. Of course, it turned out that it *was* breast cancer, not lung cancer. They sequenced her DNA to identify exactly what sort of chemo would work, found the artery that fed the tumours in her breast and put the chemo through a tube inserted in her inner thigh that ran through the body up to the artery itself. This meant they didn't have to blast her whole body with it. They managed to shrink both the breast and brain tumour she'd developed, and give her months more life, so she was able to spend quality time with her grandson Asa after he was born.

Challenging the status quo

Unbelievable, isn't it, how different the approach was? This was over ten years ago, and although I can't be certain, of course I've always thought that if we'd gone to Germany first off, my mum would still be alive today. Or it would have been even better to know about the different treatments offered in different countries! I was stonewalled at every turn. And my mother-in-law, who died at the end of 2023, also had an awful time. She wasn't misdiagnosed – she had bone cancer – but there was no talk of protecting her immune system with food or vitamin supplements. She couldn't have the stem-cell therapy she needed because the local centre had shut down. She'd had all the usual chemo, antibiotics, loads of stress on her system, so her body's defences were on the floor. I was like, *You're joking* – I couldn't believe the doctors weren't focusing on building her immunity to counter the negative impacts of the treatment. To be honest, it was also a real challenge to get people to listen to me; after all, I'm not a doctor!

I hate the 'they know best' deference. Nowadays, so many more of us are able to educate ourselves on our health so that we can advocate for ourselves when we need to. This is absolutely brilliant, and I'm a firm believer that knowledge is power! This idea that every single doctor knows everything that's out there is crazy. I'm not dumping on our doctors at all – I think they do a really tough job in difficult circumstances. I'm grateful for our health service. But if every doctor knows the same information, then why are treatments in other countries different? In fact, why are there different treatments available in different postcodes in the UK? If it was all 'correct', everyone would do the same thing, surely? Why do we attack disease with treatments where the side effects can be even more dangerous than what's being treated in the first place? Why is the DNA sequencing that I was told a decade ago wouldn't help my mum now on offer over here? Because medical thinking and research moves on, and there's nothing wrong with having an enquiring mind and seeking a second opinion. But so many of us just accept what we're told, even when our lives are on the line. We are taught from an early age to comply; and when we are scared, this becomes even more automatic. It can just feel too big for us to deal with, so we freeze and don't look for a second opinion.

I do not want my children to go through what I went through, listening to their mum beg them to end her life. I want to know what I can learn from this to save my dad from the same fate, and what I can do to help myself. What I'm discovering is that we can all put things in place not just to futureproof our own health, but for the next generations, too.

The research time lag

It's also worth pointing out that what we're being told *now* by the big healthcare providers is not the most up-to-date information. Studies have shown that on average, there's a seventeen-year time lag in 'translational research'.[4] What this means is that all the innovative and interesting medical research that's happening *right now*, won't trickle down to become advice your GP gives you for another seventeen years! Within the medical community, this is called the time lag from 'bench to bedside'.

But the great news is, we don't need to wait any more. There are so many doctors, scientists and naturopaths now, like Dr David Sinclair, Dr Peter Attia and Dr Nasha Winters, to name but a few, who are sharing all this, through social media posts, books, podcasts, academic papers and interviews. You don't need to just take my word for it, everything here is based on real experts conducting real research, not tin-hatty conspiracy crap! We can challenge the assumptions and the 'this is how we do it' orthodoxy of so much of the medical establishment – I have found that the future is looking really hopeful and positive.

In 2024, Macmillan Cancer Support conducted analysis that highlighted that cancer survival rates in the UK are as much as twenty-five years behind the rest of Europe.[5] A little-known fact but one that will mean life and death to millions and makes me even more passionate about fighting for more advanced and targeted approaches. At the Health Optimisation Summit, I learned about so many new and exciting cancer treatments that reminded me of how much we are still learning and how important it is for us to have a handle on these developments so we can advocate for ourselves and our families. I was particularly intrigued about IV therapy, hyperthermia treatment, diet interventions (specifically the keto diet and limiting pesticide exposure), metronomic immunotherapy and use of acupuncture.

Looking at our health as a whole

I found a great quote from the late Dr Mark Boguski, who was an expert in human disease genes. He said, 'What we call good medicine is doing what works for most of the people most of the time, but not everyone is most people.' I agree. There's so much exciting work looking at the future of personalised healthcare and treating the body as a whole. Now, I hate the word 'holistic' as it can sound a bit woo-woo, which, as you know, is not me at all! But holistic really does just mean 'the whole'; an understanding that disease doesn't come out of nowhere, it's a symptom of what's going on in the rest of our body and our wider environment.

Someone else who inspires me is Dr Nasha Winters, a naturopathic doctor and cancer specialist. She's popularised the term 'terrain' to describe what we should be focusing on. In essence, she says that if you successfully get rid of your cancer through chemo or drugs, you should then look at the 'terrain' of your life and improve all areas of your lifestyle that could aid your chances of recovery. For example, if you were a smoker before, it would make sense to replace that habit with a healthier one. In her approach, she sees cancer as a symptom, so you need to change the wider terrain of the body – just look at the lymph glands, the vein system, never mind the nervous system, everything is linked! And you need to change the terrain *now*, because if you get ill, the last thing you'll want to do is change the habits of a lifetime when you're lying in a hospital bed and someone's offering to get you a Subway and a Coke from the on-site canteen.

Why it's not 'just my genes'

A common response I hear a lot when it comes to disease and ageing is 'Oh well, there's nothing I can do about it, it's in my genes to get diabetes/breast cancer/dementia.' In fact, research increasingly shows us that our genes aren't the be-all-and-end-all. You might have heard lots of chat in recent years about *epigenetics* – it's one of those words that seems to have crossed over into the mainstream, but lots of us aren't sure what it actually means. Epigenetics is amazing because it shows us more and more that we are *not* entirely pre-destined by our genetic inheritance.

Put simply – because honestly, I need a straightforward explanation as much as the next person – our genetics are the DNA we inherit from our parents. But, and this is what's incredible, not all our DNA code gets 'switched on'. That's where epigenetics comes in, which was a field of science first popularised by a doctor called Bruce Lipton – someone I have had the privilege of hanging out with, once at a longevity conference in the Maldives and then again at a far less glamorous convention in rainy Manchester. In the late 1980s he carried out an experiment with skin cells in petri dishes, proving it was their environment which determined whether they would turn into muscle, bone or fat, not their genetic coding.

'Epi' means 'above' and basically refers to the environment and lifestyle choices that tells our DNA how to behave. Epigenetics explains why identical twins – people with exactly the same genes – can have different weights or have different health issues. It's their *lifestyle choices* that result in different expressions of the same genes. What's more, by studying twins, research has shown that only *25 per cent* of the difference in lifespan is down to genetics. The rest is down to what we do. This has massive repercussions for the rest of us.

Experts have come up with different metaphors to explain the difference between genetics and epigenetics: that DNA loads the gun, but lifestyle pulls the trigger, that DNA is the hardware and our epigenome is the software, that DNA is a piano with a set number of keys, but there are an infinite number of ways we can create music from it . . . the list goes on! It is important to note here that we cannot influence all of our genetic inheritance. For example, we cannot 'switch off' the BRCA gene; however, it is true that we have more influence over our health destiny than previously thought.

16

The exciting part of this is that epigenetics shows us that we do have some control, even though we can't control the genes we're born with. What we put in our mouth, do with our body, the environment we live in – all these things play a massive part in how our genes get expressed. Importantly, this links back to those diseases like cancer and dementia – they're not down to just your inherited genes, but rather the results of changes to our epigenome. And it's not all bad news. On the positive side, recent research shows that a healthy lifestyle – not smoking, being active, eating and sleeping well – can mitigate the impact of life-shortening genes by 60 per cent, giving you up to five years more of life.[6] Mind-blowing!

What this book will do for you

I've called this book *Futureproof,* because it's a full body MOT for you, to ensure that you have a vital, healthy life. It's *Futureproof* because I want *all* of us to look towards the future as something full of hope and joy, not something we've blanked out because the prospect is too bleak. It's *Futureproof* because there are so many brilliant new discoveries out there right now, like tests and tech and wearables, that will help us look after ourselves and change our health for the better.

Through hacks, advice and protocols, we're going to treat the hallmarks of ageing as a disease, not as the inevitable. **You'll be able to lower inflammation, build muscle, eat well, improve mental energy and mobility, reduce stress and feel fantastic**. We'll enjoy our lives to the full, and so when the time comes for us to leave this planet, it'll be like a Hollywood movie – not an action movie where we're thrown across a room, but a nice, gentle romcom where we drift away peacefully, preferably in our sleep and not on mind-bending painkillers.

The reality around us might be worrying, but we have the solution already. So, let's get on it, us regular, everyday people who refuse to put our heads in the sand any more. Let's rip the plaster off, look at what we can do, and futureproof our next few decades from avoidable harm.

Dealing with the critics

Those of you who follow me on Instagram have probably already read a lot of the criticism that gets thrown my way. Honestly, I've heard it all before: *you're not a doctor, relax and have fun, life's too short, you only live once!*

Let's address that first issue – I don't *want* to be a doctor, thank you very much! They seem to be in an impossible situation at the moment. I want to be able to read, interview and ask the experts who are conducting all this brilliant research from a layperson's point of view. One of the fantastic things about the time we live in is that everything is accessible; we can read or listen to the latest academic research about ageing when we're on our morning commute. Not only that, but by nature I am very non-conformist, so I wouldn't last long in any industry that expected me not to be constantly questioning the powers that be ... after all, as David Sackett, the father of evidence-based medicine said, 'Half of what you'll learn in medical school will be shown to be either dead wrong or out of date within five years of your graduation.'[7] He famously encouraged doctors to keep learning, so surely a little bit of questioning is a good thing?!

As I said, it seems like a hard time to be part of the medical establishment. It was clear during the 2024 US election campaign that health is becoming an increasingly important political issue that voters are more and more vocal about. Now, I'm not one for political debate, but I'm definitely pleased to see more people questioning bodies like the FDA (the US Food and Drug Administration) who are responsible for the regulation of so many of the products we consume. (I recently learned that in 2021 the FDA admitted that 45 per cent of its funding comes from its own users and 75 per cent of the FDA's drug division budget is also paid for by their users. Surely this causes a conflict of interest?)[8]

What I care about most is transparency and being able to make up my own mind by looking at the facts. As a mum, I want to know that what I am bringing into our house is safe and going to make us all healthier people who will live pain and disease free for as long as possible. In this book I plan to share with you everything I have learned and found through trial and error to work for me.

And on the 'just have fun' front? This idea of what constitutes 'fun' needs to be reframed, in my opinion. We're all spoon-fed this 'mummy wine o'clock' nonsense about doing whatever we want to make us 'happy', but do you know what – it's not bloody working, is it? I'm like *hang on, let's think about this attitude, shall we?* I've had enough wine and frigging chocolate bars in my lifetime to know that it has never made me feel better afterwards. I might have got a temporary boost from the dopamine-driven anticipation, but it will always end up giving me a food hangover; a sugar crash and awful cravings for more. Now, I always fast-forward and ask myself, will this satisfy me, or will it kick off a craving for more? Not to mention being an alcoholic nearly destroyed me. I can say with confidence now that yeah, life is too short to think that *that* is a fucking treat!

Let's do this together

With this book, I urge you to open your mind. Embrace the possibility of change. Changing our beliefs about ageing, what longevity is about. Because God knows, we need it! Let's take an enquiring look at the received wisdom and apply some critical thinking to the new information out there. I want all of us to be able to carry on being as active and healthy as possible for the rest of our lives. If I want to shove on a pair of trainers and go for a run when I'm a hundred, then I should be able to! I don't think that's too much to ask.

We're all going to build resilience – become more mentally strong and physically energetic, with an optimistic outlook. And this is for all of us, not just the elite athletes, or the super-rich 1 per cent! (By the way, elite athletes die young too – so fret not, no ridiculous, unachievable exercise regime in here, either!) I'm going to share some super-effective hacks, tips and protocols so we can all live in the best health possible. Because if we're living longer, we may as well live well. What have you got to lose?

FUTUREPROOF PRINCIPLE #1: PUT OUT THE INFLAMMATION FIRE

When I was at my unhealthiest, I used to internally chastise myself for being 'lazy' and lacking willpower. It seemed that whatever I did, whatever advice I tried to follow, I couldn't get out of the cycle I was in. I would inevitably cave into 'temptation', to cravings, to hunger, and reach for sugary, carby snacks, which only made me feel worse. What I've come to learn now has flipped that perception of my so-called weakness on its head. Now I understand that I was chronically inflamed, and the cascade of health problems that came from that root cause were likely behind most of my symptoms – physical, mental and emotional. And yes, my addiction to crap foods! Looking back, my biggest problem was a lack of education around my lifestyle choices.

Inflammation really is public enemy number one when it comes to ageing us. We're seeing the consequences of it everywhere, in every single aspect of our health and wellbeing. I honestly cannot underestimate how important it is to understand chronic inflammation – and experts agree. What is hugely exciting, though, is that with this knowledge comes power. We *can* do lots about it. In this chapter I'm going to share some truly jaw-dropping facts about what chronic inflammation is, what it's doing to us, the wrong information we've been fed for years (honestly, you'll be *fewmin'*), plus the simple hacks we can ALL apply to dampen down the inflammatory fire.

WHAT IT FEELS LIKE TO BE INFLAMED

I was incredibly inflamed for many years, which had severely detrimental effects on my health. I was swollen and retaining water; around my feet, my hands, even my knees were puffy. My muscles were constantly fatigued: my legs felt heavy, lifting the kids up was hard, even loading the shopping into the back of the car was an effort (even though it wasn't as if it was a 20kg weight – it should have been easy!). I was brain-foggy and plagued with constant low-level anxiety and insecurity that made me dread even the thought of leaving the house. My self-esteem was on the *floor*; it was so bad I would tell myself I wasn't even good enough to make a lasagne properly.

When I asked my Instagram followers for their experience of inflammation, I was overwhelmed by the responses, and seeing just how much people were struggling with it. '[I feel it] all over, weight gain, sore joints, tiredness,' said Jenny. Others agree that their joints were suffering – feeling 'like [they're] hit with a hammer' said Nicola, and there didn't seem to be an area that *wasn't* affected by inflammatory pain, with hips, knees, shoulders, elbows, neck, hands, feet and even fingers all flaring up for loads of you. Digestive issues were also persistent, with Aileen explaining that she 'had a tummy that looked six months pregnant', and others like Rebecca, Alana and Denise, to name but a few, all struggling with stomach complaints. I can completely relate to Kerry's comment that her body felt 'heavy like cement' – that was me!

When I was in that awful head-and-body space, trudging around Sainsbury's and chucking Snickers and salt-and-vinegar crisps into the trolley because I craved energy, my body was actually in a high state of alert. My cells were literally on fire, inflamed and behaving as if I was under attack from invaders. I didn't know it, but my system was in crisis mode. If you're struggling with energy, feel sluggish or have water retention or extra weight you can't shift – and even if you *haven't* got weight problems – you are probably dealing with chronic inflammation, which leads to a dictionary's worth of disease, illness and ageing. Inflammation is a sign that things are very wrong, and your body is screaming *argh!*

Shockingly, the root cause of this needless inflammation appears to be the shift in our Western diet that was pushed on us from the mid-twentieth century onwards: the emergence of so-called healthy convenience foods – cheap and chemically laden ultra processed foods (UPFs).

SO, WHAT ON EARTH *IS* INFLAMMATION?

Right, I need to put this front and centre – *we need some inflammation* in our bodies to survive! Without it, we would die. It is literally our natural defence against bodily trauma and exists to protect us. I'll explain. (Doing a deep dive into what's going on with inflammation can get very technical, very quickly, so I'll try and explain the science behind this as simply as possible. And if you're a chemistry or biology expert, bear with me!)

When we have a trauma – like a cut, or an injury or an infection – an alarm goes off in our immune system, which kick-starts the inflammatory process, which is there to help us. For example, say we've fallen over, cut and broken our wrist. Inflammation clots our blood, which starts the healing process. Inflammation creates heat and pain, which stops us using that broken limb so it can heal. Inflammation creates swelling, which protects the injury while it repairs. This type of inflammation is called *acute inflammation*.

Acute inflammation is caused by damage to our cell membranes, which activates a process called *oxidation*. Oxidation is how our body kills off the invaders in our cell membranes, by essentially burning them. Our bodies are clever things, and this oxidative stress sets off a chain-reaction response, where we will just keep on speedily oxidising these bad guys until the dangerous invader has been crushed.

So, inflammation is good, right? Yes, if it happens in the right circumstances, such as the above broken wrists, or when we've got a cold, or a bug we need our body to fight off. Inflammation comes in, does its job, and bang, it goes away again. Hooray.

The problem is that many elements of our modern lives – and one huge one in particular – cause *chronic inflammation*. This is when our immune system is in a constant, confused state of inflammation when it shouldn't be. This has now been proven to lead to dozens of diseases and health problems that make us weak and ill, ageing us.[1]

WHY INFLAMMATION MAKES US FEEL CRAP

When our body is under siege from a real invader, even from something as innocuous as the common cold, our inflammatory response naturally makes us feel awful. Our temperature skyrockets, we want to lie down and go to sleep, we don't want to eat anything at all. These are all natural signs of resilience, and that inflammation is working for us because it's trying to preserve our resources.

So, feeling rough is what *should* happen with acute inflammation. Our immune response is busy oxidising the baddies, causing a chemical imbalance in our cell membranes, sending out proteins called *cytokines* to tackle what it perceives as a threat to our system. The net result of this is that we have less energy. We feel ill. Feeling pain, hot, having redness or swelling – all of this is brilliant, beautiful *acute inflammation* doing its job via our immune response.[2]

So, getting a bug once or twice a year – and always, *always* after the kids go back to school, right? – is completely natural, even though it might not feel so wonderful at the time. It's the way of the world and proves that your immune system is working. When we catch these illnesses, we need good old acute inflammation to be able to swoop in and blitz the invaders.

However, suffering with low-level chronic inflammation and thus feeling rubbish all the time – tired, bloated, with loose stools or constipated, craving sugary food, sleeping poorly, aching limbs, lack of energy – isn't how things should be. It's dangerous. It not only affects how we feel, our energy levels and our weight, but also which life-limiting diseases and illnesses we may develop.

THE HORRIFIC TRUTH ABOUT CHRONIC INFLAMMATION

We now know that most age-related diseases are down to chronic inflammation.[3] It has literally been proven beyond measure that this is the root cause of dozens and dozens of illnesses and diseases that reduce our life- and healthspan and, in many cases, can even kill us: everything from obesity to insulin resistance and type 2 diabetes, depression, bipolar disorder and multiple sclerosis. Pretty much every single autoimmune disease, from lupus to psoriasis, is caused by inflammation. If we're dealing with IBS, we're inflamed. If we have acne, we're inflamed. Chronic fatigue syndrome is caused by inflammation, as is fibromyalgia and arthritis. If we have dementia, we're inflamed. Vitiligo, eczema, Crohn's disease, PMS . . . inflammation, every single time![4] The horrifying list just goes on and on.

Inflammation is also at the root of many cancers, too. 'Cancer and inflammation are closely connected,' writes Professor Fran Balkwill, who is an expert in cancer biology[5] – indeed, scientists have known this fact for more than a hundred and fifty years! The link between chronic inflammation and cancer is so serious that Cancer Research UK has funded a huge programme of international research to get to the bottom of this.[6] Money is literally pouring into understanding the consequences of chronic inflammation from medical research all over the globe.

INFLAMMAGING – AND HOW WE CAN LEARN TO TACKLE IT

It's utterly shocking to discover that these diseases, so many of which are hallmarks of ageing, are down to the same source. In fact, the effect of chronic inflammation on our longevity is so established that it has its own term: *inflammaging*.[7]

This can all seem very depressing, can't it? OK, so now we know without a doubt that chronic inflammation makes us ill and ages us. It attacks everything from the digestive tract to our endocrine (hormone), blood sugar, musculoskeletal and immune systems. Er, brilliant!

But – and this is important – by getting to the root cause of this inflammation, we can alleviate the symptoms. We can start to repair the damage that our body is wreaking on itself. It's where the future of functional medicine is going, and some pioneering and brave scientists are publishing amazing work which I am literally devouring! It's all about looking for the targets, such as environmental factors, lifestyle choices and, most importantly, our abysmal modern diet. Rather than trying to medicate ourselves out of it with anti-inflammatory drugs (which can have all sorts of other side effects, particularly on the gut and the mood), we can tackle inflammation by looking at our *terrain* – what we're doing that enables damaging chronic inflammation to thrive all over the body.

Do I have chronic inflammation?

There are tests available which will check your blood for common inflammatory markers. Tests vary, but they can look for one or more of the following:

- *C-reactive protein:* high levels could risk heart disease and depression
- *Homocystine:* an amino acid linked to dementia, heart disease and autoimmune conditions
- *Ferritin:* elevated iron levels can be a sign of inflammation
- *Intestinal permeability:* your gut lining is a sign of how inflamed (or not) you are – we'll go into that a bit more later
- *Glucose and insulin:* these measure how resistant your cells are to insulin, a marker of inflammation – another thing we'll talk about later on in this chapter!

However fascinating these are (and I do love a test), you don't necessarily need to spend money on a blood test to determine whether you are chronically inflamed or not. If you're suffering with any of the illnesses or conditions mentioned above, you are probably inflamed. A complete list of conditions caused by inflammation can be found in Dr Cate Shanahan's book *Dark Calories.*

WHAT CAUSES CHRONIC INFLAMMATION?

As I said, extensive research has identified the culprits behind our epidemic of chronic inflammation, and there are quite a number. Everything from toxins, allergens, the health of our microbiome, infections, smoking, drinking alcohol to stress and anxiety have been cited. However, nothing has been found to be more influential than *what we eat*; not only the type of food we consume, but carrying excess weight is also a major catalyst for chronic inflammation. Dr Mark Hyman has said that our modern diet is the 'primary driver' of inflammation, thanks to its highly processed, nutrient-deficient content. This ill-prepared food, made with crap chemical ingredients, has been proven to be a toxic bomb going off inside us.

WHY VEGETABLE OIL IS PUBLIC ENEMY NUMBER ONE

If you've read my previous books, you probably remember me banging on about UPFs making us sluggish, ill, wrecking our hormonal balance and just generally being a disaster zone. So much of what we eat is complete crap. It is *not food*. I mean, I am far from the only person to point this out these days and thank God! More and more brilliant scientists and experts, like Dr Chris van Tulleken to name just one, are shouting from the rooftops about the real dangers posed by UPFs, how they are behind so much of our modern health woes, and that we should take them out of our diets.

However, it is becoming even clearer there is one ingredient – highly prevalent in UPFs – which is an absolute shitshow for our health and longevity. It is a highly, highly unstable ingredient that has been forced on us via every medium you can imagine – convenience food, baby food, 'health' food, 'treat' food, restaurant food, snacks. We've been told over the years that it is good for us, and it's so cheap that it's used everywhere. Yet we are now discovering more and more how chemically reactive it is, how poisonous for our systems, and how it literally causes our bodies to become inflamed. Yep, it's our old friend vegetable oil.

WHAT IS VEGETABLE OIL AND WHY IS IT A PROBLEM?

Despite the name, vegetable oil doesn't come from vegetables. It was originally a by-product of industrial processes that have nothing to do with food (primarily the soapmaking and animal-feed industries – *heave*). Veg oil must be heavily processed in multiple, complicated stages to make it fit for human consumption – but whether it's truly fit or not I believe is now not even up for debate! It is a million miles away from something like olive oil, which is created by squeezing the oil out of the fruit. Vegetable oils can even be used to power machinery – think of McDonald's proudly plastering the sides of their lorries with the fact it's running on old cooking oil! Yet we consume it in huge quantities. (I've discovered so much more of the horrendous truth about veg oil thanks to Dr Cate Shanahan's brilliantly researched book, *Dark Calories*, and it is shuddering stuff – I recommend this as a must-read.)

First, we need to know that all these oils listed below are types of vegetable oils (also sometimes called 'seed oils' – another pseudo-healthy, misleading name):-

- Rapeseed (sometimes called canola oil in the US)
- Sunflower
- Corn
- Cottonseed
- Safflower
- Soybean
- Rice bran

I cannot undersell just how prevalent vegetable oil is in our diets. Turn over the packaging of most ultra-processed foods and you'll see at least one of these oils listed. There aren't yet conclusive stats on the proportion of veg oil consumed in the average UK diet, but it has been found to take up an incredible 30 per cent of the calories of the average American diet. That's almost a third of their energy intake from this one ingredient alone.

To be clear, these vegetable oils are different to the brilliant fruit oils and other fats we use in food and cooking which can contribute to our health and enhance our food! Those include:

- Extra virgin olive oil (a fruit oil)
- Avocado oil (a fruit oil)
- Cold pressed sesame oil (for flavour, not for frying)
- Coconut oil
- Ghee
- Butter
- Tallow
- Goose fat
- Lard

31

ALL FATS ARE NOT CREATED EQUAL!

As well as its chemical composition, which I will explain shortly, there's another important reason why veg oil is inflammatory, and that's the type of fat it is. More facts! (Bear with me, because this is vital info, I promise.)

Veg oils are *polyunsaturated* fats. There are three types of fats, all of which we need in certain amounts. The main sources of these different fats are:-

- **Saturated fats**
  - like butter, coconut oil, beef fat, milk, cream, palm oil
- **Unsaturated fats**, which come in one of two types:
  - **monounsaturated** like olive oil, avocado/peanut oils, lard, poultry fat
  - **polyunsaturated** including vegetable oils listed above, fish/flax/sesame oils

Like I've said many times before, we need fat to live. Our bodies are literally made of the stuff! Women should have a ratio of about 21–32 per cent body fat, men about 10–20 per cent. For those of us who grew up amidst the low-fat mania of the 1980s and 90s, this is something that's difficult to get our heads around. We've been conditioned so intensely to fear fat that the idea that consuming fat is *good* can feel crazy. However, it is, but what we're increasingly seeing is just how important what *type* of fat we're eating is.

What's becoming clearer and clearer now are the detrimental effects that have come from ferociously changing our diet over the past fifty years or so, switching from one dietary fat to another. In our grandparents' generation and way back for hundreds of years before, we humans mainly ate saturated or monounsaturated fats – cooking with butter, or lard, eating the whole animal nose to tail.

However, that approach completely fell out of fashion in favour of so-called heart-healthy polyunsaturated fats in the form of vegetable oils which come in margarines, low-fat food and pretty much all UPFs. We now know there are huge problems with consuming these as our main fat source; because they are chemically unstable, reactive fats that cause our bodies to chronically inflame.

THE WORRYING ROLE OF PUFAS

All those flipping ads for low-calorie, low-fat foods, plus the global food and health markets, have told us for years that polyunsaturated fats are the 'good fats', especially in comparison to the so-called saturated fat 'baddies'. Generations of people swapped butter for margarine, and fatty cuts of meat for lean meat and low-cal ready meals, believing they were doing the right thing for their health. But this anti-fat orthodoxy that's been shoved down our throats for decades is now being shown to be complete nonsense, and in fact the reverse is true! I will get to how saturated fat and cholesterol became demonised a bit later on, but for now, we need to understand how the composition of veg oil links to inflammation.

Essential fatty acids are fats our body doesn't make and we need them in our cells, so they have to come from our diet. Inside polyunsaturated fats, you have polyunsaturated fatty acids (PUFAs). Our cells are actually made up of one-third PUFAs in their natural state, and it's there as our inbuilt alarm system. So far, so straightforward. However, there are two main types of PUFAs – omega-3 and omega-6, and they have very, very, different effects on us. Remember, not all PUFAs are created equal! Basically, omega-3 (found in food like salmon and mackerel) reduces inflammation, omega-6 fatty acids promote it. And you know what I'm going to say, don't you? Vegetable oil is full of omega-6 PUFAs.

WHAT HAPPENS WHEN WE EAT VEGETABLE OILS

The reason that the omega-6 PUFA in veg oil creates inflammation is because of its chemical structure. Unsaturated basically means it's chemically unstable and that's bad news for us, because of *oxidation,* which I covered earlier when I described how acute inflammation works. (Were you listening at the back? Good!) Pretty much the same thing happens when we eat food that's either made with, or cooked in, vegetable oil. Here's the process:-

→ Vegetable oil is heated for cooking, or used as an ingredient in food . . .
→ Because it's *unstable*, it reacts with oxygen to create new chemical compounds . . .
→ We eat it . . .
→ These cause oxidative stress to start in our cells . . .
→ Oxidative stress sounds an internal alarm in our system, kick-starting the inflammation process to get rid of the 'invader' . . .
→ The process keeps going, oxidising the polyunsaturated

fatty acids in our cell membranes until they're done . . .
→ And congratulations, we are now chronically inflamed!

We can't change how our bodies respond to these PUFAs. Your poor system can't tell the difference between a real invader like a virus or a wound and a bag of crisps fried in veg oil. All it knows is that it needs to keep oxidising these fatty acids until they're gone, putting our cells under constant oxidative stress which stops them from working properly.

A great analogy, which I've borrowed from Dr Cate, is to think about a tree in a forest. The tree's wood isn't harmful until oxygen and heat combine once it's set alight, creating dangerous smoke. Our bodies catch fire when they start to oxidate the unstable veg oils, creating chemical compounds which are highly toxic and spark inflammation.

When you boil it down to the brass tacks, the cascade of consequences is simple:

unstable vegetable oil → heat → oxidation → oxidative stress → inflammation → disease

It is staggering that so much of our diet, and especially pre-prepared, processed foods, are absolutely crammed with PUFAs. By eating them, we're putting our poor bodies under constant oxidative stress and perpetuating the cycle of chronic inflammation. Being in a constant state of oxidation damages our DNA, our protein and our lipids. It also deprives our body of *antioxidants*, which are there to help us reduce unnecessary inflammation. Argh!

HOW PUFAS CREATE INFLAMMATORY BODY FAT

Eating a diet crammed full of PUFAs has also been shown to change the type of fat we have in our bodies. Back in the days where we ate proper food, up until the mid-twentieth century, the percentage of our body fat that was made up of PUFAs was between 3 and 5 per cent. The latest figures from 2008 – and let's be frank, they've probably gone up even more by now – show that it had risen to 25–30 per cent. Because of this radical change in the type of fat we eat, we now have a different biological composition.

Now, I can hear you asking, *why is this important?* Why does it matter if our fat is broken down into different percentage components than it was a hundred years ago? Simply put, because it puts us into a different metabolic state than before. Having more PUFA in our body fat not only makes us flabbier (as far back as the 1980s, a doctor called John Yudkin was noticing that PUFA fat is looser and less solid than saturated fat body weight) but it is more prone to inflammation.

WHY INFLAMMATORY FAT CAN LEAD TO INSULIN RESISTANCE

Having more inflammatory body fat slows down our ability to generate energy from the food we consume – what we call our *metabolism*. Having an excess of inflamed body fat can disrupt how our bodies convert food into usable energy (metabolism). Because this inflamed fat impairs normal energy production, the body often compensates by pulling more glucose out of the bloodstream. This can cause dips in blood sugar that trigger sugar cravings, perpetuating a cycle of overeating and blood-sugar swings.

Over time, the chronic elevation of blood sugar and inflammation can lead to insulin resistance – a condition in which the body's cells become less responsive to insulin. Insulin resistance is a common precursor to type 2 diabetes and is associated with a host of other health issues. It also makes maintaining a healthy weight more difficult because cells that don't respond well to insulin struggle to access energy, causing continued fatigue and cravings, all while promoting further fat accumulation.

And it's not just something that may affect you if you're overweight. You can have a so-called 'healthy' body-fat percentage but still be massively inflamed and insulin resistant if a high proportion of the fat you do have is made up of PUFAs. This is why the crude tests you get at the GP (e.g. BMI test) are so unhelpful; they're just looking at one basic measurement and using that to tell you if you're OK or not. But it's simply not true! You can be slim but still carrying loads of inflammatory visceral body fat around your organs, which can be just as dangerous.

WE'VE GOT 'HEALTHY EATING' ALL WRONG

Right now, horribly, it looks as if people around my age will be the first generation to live longer than their children. Younger generations are growing up so unhealthily that they're headed for life-limiting disease. Stats show that those born from the 1990s onwards are three times more likely to be obese compared with their parents or grandparents.[8] Generational lifespan is decreasing – and in our so-called modern society, where we are supposed to be more evolved and knowledgeable than ever before. Instead, we are at a crisis point!

We need to take a hard look at the 'healthy eating' advice we're being given, because it's clearly not working. The softly-softly approach of 'just have everything in moderation', the US food pyramid, the NHS's Eatwell plate, the millions of pounds spent on promoting Five a Day . . . None of this has fixed our issues so far, has it? In fact, things have got much, much worse. Adult obesity rates in the UK have risen from 15 per cent in 1993 to 28 per cent now,[9] and 23 per cent of eleven-year-old kids in the UK are obese – that's almost a quarter. Globally, obesity is a huge crisis – rates have tripled since the 1970s – and it's linked to increased risks of many diseases.[10]

IT'S NOT ABOUT FAT-SHAMING!

I want to be completely clear: I am not fat-shaming *anyone* here. My focus is the complete opposite. If you are struggling with your weight, which is something I did for many, many years, you can feel utterly hopeless, especially if you're doing everything you've been told is 'right' and still nothing changes. So I'm not blaming us for this mess – I'm furious at the food manufacturers. When vegetable oils have been sold to us as the 'healthy' alternative to saturated fats, no wonder so many of us are in a constant state of chronic inflammation and dealing with excess weight! (Oh, and if you read my last book, *Hack Your Hormones*, you'll know that veg oils suppress leptin, the satiety hormone that tells us we've had enough to eat. So, as well as inflaming us, we're also left absolutely starving. It's a total catch-22!)

We only need to look around us to know that something is very wrong with public health, and it appears to have its roots in when we shifted our diets from consuming natural, saturated fat to heavily processed polyunsaturated vegetable oils. When I was growing up, convenience foods were taking over, but there was at least the echo of our grandparents' generation who cooked from scratch with real ingredients. I mean, I absolutely *hated* them at the time, but at least we had things like stews! I look back and think now, at least it was deep nutrition, rather than what we do now, which is chucking out two millenniums' worth of human knowledge about what our bodies need in favour of using bloody Vitalite!

INFLAMMATION = INSIDE EMERGENCY

Remember, a third of our cells are naturally PUFA for a reason – in case of an emergency such as infection. But by eating a diet full of PUFAs, we are turning our bodies into a 24/7 emergency zone. Chronic inflammation is causing chaos inside us, it's making us feel like crap and it's reducing our healthspan.

But things are changing. Pioneering scientists and medics are now revealing the truth about the root causes of chronic inflammation and how it is fundamentally killing us. However, Rome wasn't built in a day, and we need to start somewhere. First, we need to begin by unravelling our diets from the life-limiting poison that is vegetable oils.

TACKLING INFLAMMATION #1 – TAKE OUT VEG OIL

Vegetable oil really is the absolute worst, and if there's one thing you should do to reduce chronic inflammation, it's to take this toxic ingredient out of your diet.

First up, the good news. It's not going to be as hard as it could be. Take it from me, I've white-knuckled my way through coming off first alcohol, then sugar and refined carbs, and at points it's been grim. But the difference with veg oil is that your palate's not going to miss it! It's completely tasteless (because it's been bleached and deodorised, ugh). So hooray, hooray, it's probably one of the easiest foods ever to eliminate, because you will not be craving it. There's no chance you'll be thinking *Oh God, I'm desperate for some vegetable oil* in the same way you might crave a pizza.

Even better, you're replacing it with something more delicious. Butter, olive and avocado oils are all easily available and taste lovely. There's no white knuckling involved. However, although it's easy enough to swap out the cooking oil you use at home, the challenge with veg oil is checking the foods that it has sneaked into without you even realising. It has made its evil little way into thousands of items we all consume unwittingly. If you are reading this at home, go to your cupboard right now, choose five items and check the ingredients list for vegetable oil.

But do not worry – I've got your back. Towards the end of this chapter, I've put together a list of easy swaps you can make next time you're at the supermarket or online grocery shopping, plus how to read misleading labels as well as a list of the absolute worst ingredients to avoid so you can reduce your inflammatory response.

Aren't other things worse for us than veg oil?

To be quite honest, I would rather you have a block of (vegetable oil free) chocolate as a treat, rather than consume any vegetable oil. I'm not kidding! Now, I'm not saying for a moment that sugary foods, or even alcohol for that matter, are good for inflammation – they're not. In fact, both are known to cause an inflammatory response. But it's about which should be our priority focus. The reason I focus on vegetable oil is that it seems to be the real gateway to overeating, at least for me.

Let's look at alcohol first. Of course, there is no 'safe' level of alcohol consumption and, as a recovering alcoholic, I know this more than most. As well as addiction, alcohol is linked to all sorts of inflammatory conditions like fatty liver disease. And we all know how difficult it is to resist snacking on crisps or ice-cream once we've had a couple of glasses and our blood sugar is all over the place!

So, it's never 'good' for you, no matter what all those articles claim are the health benefits of a glass of red wine a night. I mean, come on, who ever restricted themselves to one small glass? Not me. In some ways, I feel lucky to be an alcoholic, because drinking is just completely off the table for me, so I don't have to deal with the temptation of stopping early! I really think the messaging around alcohol (moderation) isn't helping people: it is a highly addictive substance, FFS! No wonder so many of us struggle with it.

Sugary foods, and especially the added sugars present in UPFs, are also terrible for inflammation – plus they're known to promote overeating and reduce our satiety levels. (If you want more of a deep dive into how these ultra-processed foods completely mess with our hormone response, then I'd recommend reading the 'Why Can't I Stop Eating?' chapter in my last book, *Hack Your Hormones*.) Both alcohol and carby foods convert to glucose in the bloodstream, and these days we are well versed in their damaging effects. After all, cancer cells are caused by the fermentation process in our cells, because tumours primarily need glucose to grow and thrive.

However! What's completely shocking, and this is something Cate Shanahan covers in *Dark Calories*, is the fact that **veg oil looks as if it's more inflammatory than sugar**. She writes about a study that showed how vegetable oil led to insulin resistance (the precursor of diabetes which we just covered) more than fructose, a type of sugar.[11] She also points out that, overall, sugar consumption in America has actually reduced during the past twenty years (which might be down to the increased use of sweeteners). Yet during the same time period, obesity rates have *doubled*. This just doesn't make sense if sugar is public enemy number one. 'In the which-is-worse contest between sugar and vegetable oil . . . vegetable oil wins hands down,' Dr Cate writes.

Look, I'm not saying that as long as you cut out veg oil you can carry on boozing and chucking sweets down your throat all day long. Of course not! But I do think we need to reframe our perceptions. Our livers process one unit of alcohol per hour, and after a few weeks without drinking at all, fatty liver inflammation is non-existent.[12] Vegetable oil hangs around in our system for five years . . . gulp gulp. However, good news, you can be free of the low mood and brain fog overnight when you cut it out!

We need to take out our addictions in the order that they're causing us harm. I took out alcohol first, because it was going to kill me if I didn't, and then I tackled sugar and carbs. With what I know now, I should have taken out vegetable oil second, as I have a feeling coming off sugar might have been easier without vegetable oil in my brain too – but do you know what, you can learn from my mistakes!

If we're trying to make achievable, long-lasting changes in our diet to improve our healthspan and overall longevity, I would recommend cutting out veg oil as a vital first step, before anything else.

INFLAMMATION AND THE MICROBIOME

Our gut microbiome plays a central role in our immune system and overall resilience to disease. Our microbiota are the millions of bacteria that live in the gut and absolutely *tons* has been written about this topic over the past few years. Unless you've been living under a rock, you'll know that promoting a healthy gut microbiome has become a super-fashionable wellness trend and we're now surrounded by products and supplements that claim to look after our gut health and promote good bacteria.

The gut microbiome *is* extremely important; it affects everything from our hormone balance to our energy levels and mental health. Most of our immune system is based in our gut, too, so if that is out of whack, which it very easily can be, chronic inflammation can run riot. We already know that things like steroids and antibiotics are a disaster zone for our microbiome, blitzing all the good bacteria and promoting the growth of harmful ones. Alcohol, too, is a bit like a hand sanitiser; it kills all the gut bacteria – hence why you feel flatline the morning after drinking! Now we're coming to understand just why our crappy modern diet wrecks it too and leads to inflammation. It's all because of leaky gut.

HOW OUR MICROBIOME RELATES TO LEAKY GUT

Now, some doctors claim there's no such thing as leaky gut, but there is something called 'increased intestinal permeability'. Er, they're the same thing! When we talk about leaky gut we're literally talking about *this* – the fact that the integrity of our gut lining can be compromised. The lining of our intestinal tract – our gut – which runs from our mouth all the way down to our bum, is super thin. It's what's known as *semipermeable*, which basically means that water, and nutrients like amino acids, fatty acids and sugars can permeate from our gut into our bloodstream, which is where they need to go. However, it keeps other harmful chemicals and toxins, like undigested food proteins, firmly within the gut thanks to its strong barrier.

With leaky gut – sorry, 'increased intestinal permeability' – the gaps between the cells in our gut lining get bigger. Instead of being semipermeable, they become *hyperpermeable*, which means molecules that shouldn't escape our gut barrier do. They flood our bloodstream and thereby activate our immune system, which is going 'Oh no, what's this?' End result? Inflammation, naturally!

Vegetable oils and chemical additives present in our UPF-heavy modern diet are highly abrasive to our gut lining. We are taking in industrialised ingredients that aren't even supposed to be in the food chain (remember where veg oil comes from?) and they are damaging our precious intestinal tract. So, looking after our gut microbiome is not just about increasing bacterial diversity, but also maintaining our gut lining's integrity. A really robust gut lining means a robust immune system that isn't compromised by chronic inflammation.

How do I know if I have leaky gut?

Leaky gut is so intertwined with chronic inflammation that many of its symptoms are the same – such as bloating, puffiness, digestive problems like IBS and Crohn's, fatigue. There is lots you can do to resolve these symptoms which we'll cover in this book, but if you want to know whether leaky gut is your issue, there are blood tests available (though not yet through the NHS) which can check for certain markers:

- *MMP-9:* this stands for matrix metalloproteinase-9 (rolls off the tongue, doesn't it?) and elevated levels are linked with increased intestinal impermeability[13]
- *Zonulin:* a group of proteins which regulate our gut permeability[14]

TACKLING INFLAMMATION #2 –
INTERMITTENT FASTING (IF)

The second step we can take to tackle chronic inflammation and restore the health of our gut microbiome at the same time is through intermittent fasting (IF). Because it's not just what we eat, but *when* we eat, too, that matters. Put simply, intermittent fasting is giving your body a break from eating for specific time periods, whether that's a day each week, or for a few hours each day.

A bit like how everyone talks about the gut microbiome nowadays, IF has crossed over into the mainstream these past few years, and for good reason! It has been proven scientifically to have real health benefits. A recent study at the University of Southern California (USC) even found that a 'fasting mimicking diet', where participants didn't actually fully fast, but simply reduced their food intake for five days a month, resulted in less inflammation and a lowered biological age.[15] And this was after only a handful of months on the plan!

There are loads of different IF plans out there – the 5:2 plan and 16:8 being the best known – but you can easily create your own. I went through how to introduce time-restricted eating in my previous books, especially in *Hack Your Hormones* as a way of managing and regulating your appetite hormones, but research has found it is absolutely incredible for improving longevity as well.

This is because whenever we eat, we kick-start the inflammatory process – even if we're not eating crappy foods! Even eating good food like an organic roast dinner will cause some level of inflammation as our bodies dive into action to digest the food. It's a major operation and bodily function to break down what we eat into its composite nutrients and move it around the body.

THE AMAZING BENEFITS OF AUTOPHAGY

Autophagy literally means 'self-eating', which sounds disgusting, but it's actually essential for our cells' health. Basically, it gives our cells a bit of a spring clean and the chance to get rid of all the nasties. Autophagy increases not only our cells' function, but also their lifespan. It allows the body to go into a state of repair and begin a vital recycling process where it clears out old crappy cells and breaks them down so that new ones can grow. Dr Mark Hyman gives a great analogy of autophagy being a bit like the old Pac-Man video game, with the little smiley face eating up all the dodgy old proteins so that new ones can form!

If we never give our bodies a chance to enter autophagy, we end up constantly inflamed – and we already know what a disaster zone that is for our health. Research has shown that autophagy is essential for maintaining a healthy gut microbiome and immune response as well.[16] This is what we want! We want to kick off this autophagic response and give our cells the chance to recuperate, recycle and replenish. To maintain a robust gut lining and reduce inflammation. So restricting our eating window to within a certain number of hours each day is a great way to manage this – and the study I mentioned above found that fasting accelerated autophagy.

You can introduce IF in loads of different ways, whatever is right for you. Depending on your preference, you could either push back your first meal of the day until later (so eating all your meals between 11 a.m. and 7 p.m., for example) or starting and finishing earlier (e.g. eating between the hours of 7 a.m. and 3 p.m.). If you follow me on Instagram, you probably know already that I tend not to eat until the afternoons and instead power myself through on a 'fat fast' with keto coffee in the mornings – more on keto below. And since going to the Lanserhof longevity clinic in Germany, I've learned about how you can promote autophagy even while consuming a small amount of fatty calories. That's now my plan for every Monday from now on – to give my cells a good clean-out! I'll chat more about this in the chapter on Futureproof Principle #3: Eat for Vitality.

You'll know yourself how sluggish you end up feeling when you're snacking in the office all day. Instead, I'd recommend having a tablespoon of MCT oil which will stop you feeling hungry, whilst avoiding kicking off the digestive system. (MCT, in case you haven't read my previous books and are wondering what I'm talking about, stands for 'medium-chain triglyceride.) This protocol will keep you in autophagy and keep you energised. It's a win–win!

In the back of this book, in the **Futureproof Living section**, I'll set out a step-by-step way to introduce IF if you want to follow a plan. The important thing is that we give our bodies a rest and allow this amazing process to work its anti-inflammatory magic.

TACKLING INFLAMMATION #3 – KETOGENIC DIET (KETO)

The keto diet is actually more than 100 years old. It was first used as a treatment for epilepsy after a doctor saw that it reduced seizures in many of his patients. Basically, the keto diet is a low-carbohydrate, high-fat eating plan designed to shift the body into a state called *ketosis.*

In ketosis, the body primarily burns fat for fuel instead of carbohydrates. When you limit your carb intake, the liver produces ketones, which are molecules created from the breakdown of fats. These ketones serve as an alternative energy source for the brain and body. Essentially, a keto diet aims to induce and maintain this metabolic state, encouraging fat utilisation for energy and potentially leading to weight loss.

One of the main ways keto can help reduce inflammation is by increasing our metabolic response. We've already covered how eating too many PUFAs increases our inflammatory body-fat composition, which slows down our metabolism and can lead to insulin resistance. The same happens when we eat too many refined carbs, in things like bread, pasta and wholegrains. More and more experts in the field are now advocating a keto-style approach, cutting down on carbs and increasing consumption of good fats. This is not only for weight loss, but also because it appears to have numerous long-term health benefits, too.

THE LONGEVITY BENEFITS OF KETO

Keto is now being talked of as a new way of managing – and reversing – type 2 diabetes. Science journalist Gary Taubes has been writing for years about reducing carbohydrate consumption as a protocol for both obesity and diabetes (which as we know, are both caused by inflammation). In his latest book, *Rethinking Diabetes,* he describes carbs as a 'poison', because they are converted immediately into blood glucose, leading to too much insulin production and, over time, insulin resistance.

His position is that diabetics should follow a low-carb diet, to manage their condition and get them off drugs like metformin.

Another study done in the UK by a forward-thinking local GP called Dr David Unwin showed that a low-carb diet actually reversed type 2 diabetes in more than half of the patients that followed it![17] Similar research done in the US demonstrated the same. And when type 2 diabetes rates are soaring – doubling in this country since 2005 – this is heartening to see.

There are also studies that show keto can help as a treatment for breast cancer[18] – the low-carb, high-fat focus lowers levels of blood glucose. So far, keto is only being promoted as an additional treatment alongside conventional medicine, but the evidence is clear – keto is anti-tumour, helps the efficacy of chemo and prolongs survival. Keto has also been shown to improve cognition in Alzheimer's sufferers and has incredible impacts on mental illness, with psychiatrists successfully using it for patients with schizophrenia.

Dr Nasha Winters, the fantastic naturopathic doctor I mentioned earlier, is a big proponent of the keto diet. When I spoke to her about why, she told me that 'adopting a ketogenic or ketone body-inducing diet offers profound therapeutic po-tential in the prevention, support and even treatment of cancer by addressing the metabolic vulnerabilities of cancer cells. By reducing glucose and insulin levels, enhancing mitochondrial function and promoting metabolic flexibility, this approach empowers the body's innate healing mechanisms while tar-geting cancer's Achilles' heel – its reliance on glucose. A keto-leaning lifestyle isn't just a diet; it's a transformative tool that shifts the terrain toward resilience, creating an en-vironment less hospitable to cancer and more conducive to vibrant health.'

Recent research suggests that a ketogenic diet may help reduce relapse in some individuals with alcohol use disorder. When the liver breaks down alcohol, it produces acetate, which the brain can use for energy – particularly in chronic heavy drinkers. This shift toward relying on acetate is thought to contribute to withdrawal symptoms once drinking stops.

Ketone bodies (β-hydroxybutyrate, acetoacetate and acetone) can also serve as an alternative fuel for the brain, potentially easing the transition away from alcohol-derived acetate. Early studies indicate that people receiving treatment for alcohol addiction who follow a ketogenic diet may experience fewer withdrawal symptoms and stronger recovery outcomes compared to those consuming a standard diet. While these findings are promising, further research is needed to confirm the diet's effectiveness and understand its long-term impact on alcohol dependence.

Another recent study showed that older people with higher levels of triglycerides (a type of fat) in their blood had a *lower risk of developing Alzheimer's disease overall*.[19] I find this absolutely staggering. Good fats in the blood can actually reduce dementia risk, yet we are all still being told to cut down on fat? Madness. And personally, I would rather die from a heart attack than suffer from the traumatic 'long goodbye' of dementia.

Not all medical experts agree on adapting a ketogenic diet, but I am constantly reading more and more studies that show tangible health and disease benefits to increasing our consumption of good fats.

One of the biggest challenges with the ketogenic protocol, though, is applying it. A strict ketogenic diet plan is where we get 70–75 per cent of our calories from fat, 20–25 per cent from protein and 5 per cent from carbohydrates. It's actually really tricky to take in that much fat in our diets – we would need to be pouring olive oil on top of every single meal to increase the fat content enough! However, research demonstrates that dramatically reducing our intake of refined carbs and increasing good fats, even if we're not on a strict keto plan, will still have positive anti-inflammatory effects.

Hang on, but what about cholesterol?

Now, I know what you're probably thinking . . . what about unhealthy cholesterol levels caused by a high fat diet? I'll get straight to the point. Cholesterol is not bad for us, and the link between it and increased risk of heart disease has now been thoroughly disproved!

Our perception of cholesterol as something dangerous to be lowered at all costs has been embedded over the past few decades by the food and medical industries. However, the narrative is so confused, many of us don't even realise we *need* cholesterol. Cholesterol is an essential, waxy-like substance in the bloodstream, which plays a whole host of important roles. It helps produce our cell membranes, regulate numerous hormones, produce our bile acids and maintain our immune system. Without cholesterol we would be a puddle of liquid.

There is a whole book's worth of information behind the cholesterol health scare (and indeed, a Scottish doctor called Malcolm Kendrick has written one; it's called *The Great Cholesterol Con*). In essence, it was based on what cardiologist Dr Aseem Malhotra calls a 'fatally flawed understanding' of cholesterol's role, and a few studies from the early twentieth century whose findings were not scientifically rigorous. Even the nutritionist who is first credited with promoting the link between saturated fat, high cholesterol and heart disease, Ancel Keys, changed his standpoint, saying in 1997, 'There is no connection whatsoever between cholesterol in food and cholesterol in blood.'

Modern medicine's obsession with lowering cholesterol at all costs by demonising saturated fat may have even led to an *increase* in heart disease and obesity, by encouraging people to eat low-fat, high-carb pseudo-food UPFs instead, full of veg oils.[20] This has been an utter waste of time, lives and money. Replacing saturated fats with vegetable oils does not result in a lower risk of death from cardiovascular disease[21] and studies also show there is no significant association between cardiovascular disease and high cholesterol levels.[22] Even the American Heart Association has completely reversed their position, declaring in 2015 that cholesterol is 'no longer a nutrient of concern' for overconsumption.[23]

As I understand it, our LDL cholesterol (bad cholesterol) level can't give us the full picture of our health. Low LDL cholesterol alone will not protect you from cardiovascular issues if your insulin, glucose, hs-CRP, oxidative stress, waist circumference and triglycerides are high. Equally, high cholesterol – provided all your other markers are healthy – won't necessarily impact your heart health. Cholesterol is just one piece of the metabolic puzzle!

As you know, I'm not a scientist, but this information has stunned me because it flies in the face of the received wisdom we have all been completely bathed in since birth. And despite these fascinating findings that appear to debunk the cholesterol myth, most GPs will hold on to the lower-cholesterol-for-a-healthy-heart rhetoric like a religion!

HOW I INCORPORATE KETO INTO MY EVERYDAY

As I mentioned, maintaining strict keto in the long term can be a big challenge. The goal is not to be fully ketogenic but metabolically flexible, so we can dip in and out of carbs if we want to (as you may know, I'm a fan of my sourdough and cheese!) 'Metabolically flexible' means the body can switch from fat-burning to glucose-burning really nimbly – it's not about being in constant ketosis. We need to get our insulin levels back to an even keel and reduce inflammation, so we should avoid anything that will overly spike our blood sugar. This is what I might do on an average day:

- Morning – keto coffee with collagen and MCT oil (often more than one!). The fats in MCT oil and the amino acids in the collagen powder feed my brain so I don't need to use willpower to crush cravings
- Late lunch – scrambled eggs with mushrooms, smoked salmon, avocado – full of good fats, helping me manufacture my hormones and stay balanced!
- Afternoon snack – Greek yogurt with chocolate bone broth protein, and activated nuts
- Evening meal – roast dinner or steak and eggs with veg and bread, chocolate dessert

TOP TEN KETO-FRIENDLY SWAPS

Avocado, eggs and red meat are all staples on a keto-eating plan – plus eggs and meat are good sources of protein, which we will do a deep dive into later in this book. To get started, though, here's a quick list of easy swaps to make your diet more keto-friendly. (Not all vegetables and nuts are OK on keto as they may be high-carb. It's quite a surprise when you look into it!)

Swap	For
1. Breaded fish/chicken	Salmon or chicken thighs (with the skin on!)
2. Sweetcorn	Green beans
3. Roast potatoes	Roast aubergine/cauliflower/peppers
4. Sweetened oat milk	Cream
5. Cashews and pistachios	Pecans, almonds or walnuts (activated)
6. Sweetened, low-fat fruit yogurt	Plain full-fat Greek yogurt
7. Bananas and apples	Raspberries and strawberries
8. Diet fizzy drinks	Sparkling water with sugar-free electrolytes
9. Milk chocolate	Dark chocolate (at least 70 per cent cocoa)

HOW TO REDUCE INFLAMMATION ON YOUR WEEKLY SHOP

So far, we've covered the three main protocols for reducing inflammation, which are:

- Eliminating vegetable/seed oils
- Introducing intermittent fasting
- Reducing refined carbs, and adding in keto-friendly foods

As you know, I'm always going to promote eating whole foods rather than something that's been made in a factory. The rule of thumb is something that your grandparents would recognise as food or as a cooking ingredient. But of course, I'm not a maniac and I live in the real world.

Some days we just cannot be arsed making meals from scratch, because we're exhausted or too busy or the kids are nagging at us, or we're just *done* with all this shit for the day, and that's completely fine. None of us are perfect and we have to adapt all this information and advice into our lives. I want to make this as easy and straightforward for you – not something you end up feeling is yet another impossible chore to incorporate into your everyday.

So, this last part of the inflammation section will arm you with the information you need to have in your back pocket next time you're in the supermarket or putting together an online grocery order. The goal is to reduce our exposure to inflammation-spiking ingredients. We'll do this by:

- Deciphering the health claims made on food labels
- Understanding how to read the ingredients list
- Identifying the top five worst inflammation-causing ingredients to avoid
- Comparing and contrasting some everyday processed foods

LABEL HEALTH CLAIMS TO WATCH OUT FOR

So many claims are made about the health benefits of foods which are complete crap. For years, we consumers have been led down the garden path by clever marketing and packaging that tells us we're making a healthy choice, whereas in reality we're making anything but! So many of these phrases and slogans are not all they're cracked up to be, and we all need to be aware that we shouldn't take them at face value. Here are some of the worst offenders and what they usually mean:

Heart healthy – this generally means it's just low in saturated fat and/or cholesterol, which as we know is no marker of health. It is probably a UPF stuffed with chemical additives instead.

Low-cal – calories are not a measure of how good something is for you! We all know that not all calories are made equal, and we will likely feel hungrier and eat more after consuming low-cal UPFs rather than high-calorie natural food.

Low-fat – when food that is supposed to contain fat has been made low-fat, manufacturers will have pumped it full of inflammation-spiking ingredients to mask its absence.

Plant-based/Vegan – I've said it a thousand times already, but 'plant-based' does not equal healthy! Much plant-based food is heavily processed and full of chemical additives to mimic a meat-like taste and appearance.

One of your five a day – unless this is stuck on a piece of actual fruit or veg, approach with caution! For example, fruit juices and smoothies are a sugar bomb that lead to glucose-spiking, but we've been led to believe they're a healthy choice.

My advice is simple: next time you're at the supermarket, if you see ANY of these claims on the front of your food, I want you to do one thing. Turn it over and read the ingredients list. If there are ingredients in there you don't recognise, or any that crop up in the list below, put it back on the shelf! Brilliant – you've just saved yourself a needless dose of inflammation.

TOP TEN INGREDIENTS TO AVOID

These are the absolute worst inflammation-inducing ingredients. These are the AVOID AT ALL COSTS baddies, but it took me a long time to get there. I list them to get them on your radar because knowledge is power. Once I knew how bad these ingredients were for me, they stopped tasting as good, and gradually I cut them out. You can too!

All vegetable oils: sunflower and rapeseed are the most common
Sucralose
Aspartame
Acesulfame potassium[24] (*all three are artificial sweeteners and cause inflammatory response*)

Carrageenan
Maltodextrin[25]
Lecithin
Xanthan gum
Guar gums[26]
Any E numbers (these stabilisers, thickeners and emulsifiers
have been linked to inflammation)

LABELS LAID BARE: THE BETTER AND WORSE PROCESSED FOODS

Believe it or not, there are some processed foods out there which are a lot better for you than others. Here are just a few that I've found by popping into the supermarkets and looking at different versions of three common foodstuffs most of us will have in our kitchen: tomato soup, mayonnaise and peanut butter. It's fascinating to see how different their ingredients are, even though the product might seem the same on the surface. What's great is that it shows us it is possible to reduce inflammation even when we're buying ready-made stuff. And it's another reminder, if ever we needed one, that we should always, always read the label!

Tomato soup

INFLAMMATION SPIKING: WeightWatchers tomato soup

This soup is padded out with water, inflammatory oil and chemical additives to keep it low-calorie.
Tomato (60 per cent)
Water
Modified cornflour – *here to thicken the soup rather than use*

more tomatoes

Sugar – *a known driver of inflammation and addiction*

Salt

Dried skimmed milk

Rapeseed oil – *inflammatory oil common in so many UPFs*

Milk proteins

Sweetener – acesulfame potassium – *artificial sweetener created in a lab that is 200x sweeter than normal sugar*[27]

Spice extracts

Herb extract

Citric acid

BETTER CHOICE: Tesco tomato and basil soup with double cream

Every ingredient in this soup is something we recognise as food, and could even buy ourselves

Tomato (76 per cent) – *higher percentage of actual tomatoes than WW soup*

Tomato juice

Double cream – *natural ingredient to add richness and increase satiety*

Onion

Tomato purée

Agave syrup – *a natural sugar alternative that is OK in small amounts*

Butter – *stable, saturated fat*

Salt

Basil

Black pepper

Mayonnaise

INFLAMMATION SPIKING: Hellmann's Light Mayonnaise

Water – *hang on, isn't mayonnaise supposed to be made from mainly oil?*

Rapeseed oil (25 per cent) – *inflammatory baddy*

Spirit vinegar

Modified starch*

Sugar – *causes inflammation and addiction*

Salt

Egg yolk

Cream powder*

Citrus fibre*

Natural mustard flavouring

Thickeners – guar gum, xanthan gum* – *also known to increase pro-inflammatory cytokines*[28]

Mustard flour

Lemon juice concentrate

Antioxidant calcium disodium

Paprika extract

*all these additives are here to replace the fat that would emulsify a proper mayonnaise

BETTER CHOICE: Dr Wills Avocado Oil Mayonnaise Sugar Free

Avocado oil (76 per cent) – *saturated fat so does not provoke chronic inflammation*

Pasteurised free-range egg yolk

Water

Apple vinegar

Dijon mustard

Mustard seeds
Spirit vinegar
Salt
Lemon juice

Peanut butter

INFLAMMATION SPIKING: Tesco Stockwell & Co Crunchy Peanut Butter

Roasted peanuts (87 per cent)
Rapeseed oil – *inflammatory culprit*
Certified sustainable palm oil
Sugar – *is this really necessary?*
Salt

BETTER CHOICE: Aldi The Food Market Crunchy Peanut Butter

Peanuts (100 per cent) – *boom! That's all you need.*

What else can we do to tackle inflammation?

Oxygen Therapy

On my own journey to tackle inflammation outside of the kitchen, I have tried some weird and wonderful things. One of my favourite recent discoveries is Hyperbaric Oxygen Therapy,[29] which I am testing the benefits of in an n-of-1 study on myself collaborating with Biohacking Manchester. Hyperbaric Oxygen Therapy is a treatment that involves breathing oxygen inside a chamber that has been pressurised up to two to three times higher than standard air pressure.

These conditions allow your lungs to take in much higher levels of oxygen, which increases oxygen in your cells and tissues. In the past it has successfully been used to treat wounds that are taking a long time to heal, carbon monoxide poisoning and decompression sickness. We are still learning about all the positive benefits of increasing oxygen in the body in this way, but we know it helps to promote healing and reduce oxidative stress.

This happens because increased oxygen in our tissue is better able to fight off bad bacteria and stave off infection that causes inflammation. It also encourages new blood vessels to grow, which encourages the formation of new collagen and new skin cells.

It is accessible in some hospitals for acute treatment, but is also becoming more widely available through wellbeing clinics and at home portable HBOT chambers. My friend Dr Masha Makeeva introduced me to HBOT and has been helping me investigate this therapy for myself. I have been trying it for a few weeks and am already seeing positive results when I do long-distance running.

Nasal breathing

Perhaps a little more straightforward, I have also been focusing on nasal breathing. Now you might be thinking, *Davinia, I'm breathing through my nose right now . . . what's the big deal??* But, as it turns out, nasal breathing *is* a big deal and we're not always doing enough of it. When we're stressed, sleeping or exercising, we will often breathe through our mouths. When we do that, we are losing out on all the benefits of breathing through our noses. The principal benefits of nasal breathing are:

- Filtering out of germs, allergens, dust and other foreign particles
- Warming and moisturising the air to bring it to a comfortable body temperature that is easier for your lungs to use
- Producing nitric oxide which is a vasodilator that widens blood cells and improves blood oxygen circulation in the body

This nitric-oxide benefit is what excites me the most. As we know, more oxygen in our cells means better fighting of inflammation. As Patrick McKeown states in his book *The Oxygen Advantage*, nitric oxide has also been shown to regulate blood pressure and prevent blockages in arteries with plaque and clots. The potential impacts of this are reduced risk of heart attack and stroke, two of the top three causes of death in the UK. All it takes is breathing for the majority of the time through your nose. At night, you can make sure you do this by using mouth tape and a nose strip to open the airways. It might look a bit mad and take some getting used to, but I find I get much better sleep and wake up feeling much calmer and more relaxed. A real added benefit. You can also supplement with fermented beetroot extract if you really want to boost your nitric-oxide production. There are incredible before and after pictures of facial structure becoming more refined (strong jaw, higher cheekbones, wider smile) when we go from mouth breathing to nose breathing and hack our sleep.

MY TOP FIVE ANTI-INFLAMMATORY TAKEAWAYS

There is so much we can do to reduce inflammation, and I am passionate about spreading the word as far and wide as I can. Taking on board the knowledge that I've discovered has not only made me feel so much better, but also stronger and more resilient. On my Instagram, I've heard from so many of you who've seen and felt the benefits when you've reduced your inflammatory response. For example, Tracey, who had IBD, has seen her symptoms go into 'full remission' and has no inflammatory markers in her blood at all since ditching UPFs and following a high-protein and low-sugar diet.

We know that inflammation is a disaster zone, but we don't need to live like this. We can futureproof ourselves through education and aim for metabolic flexibility, dipping in and out of ketosis throughout the day or the week. So, try applying the top five tips below:

1. **Do not use vegetable oil!** Chuck it away and replace with olive, avocado or coconut oil, or butter.
2. **Read the ingredients lists**, and don't buy food containing the top ten nasties.
3. **Introduce intermittent fasting** in a way that suits you, to promote autophagy.
4. **Reduce refined carbs** to cut down your risk of insulin resistance.
5. **Eat more good fats** to encourage a ketogenic state.

FUTUREPROOF PRINCIPLE #2: GET STRONGER, LIVE LONGER

Right, quick quiz. What ONE thing:

- Burns fat even when you're at rest
- Balances your blood glucose levels
- Stimulates your brain function
- Protects you against disease
- Improves your metabolic health
- Cuts carb cravings
- Improves immunity
- *and* is the biggest organ in the body???

Believe it or not, the answer to all of these is our muscles! We always think that skin is the largest organ in the body, don't we? (I'm sure I was told that more than once.) But it's not – it's our amazing muscles, and I've been staggered to discover just how essential they are for maintaining longevity. When I used to think about what strong muscles meant, I – and probably lots of us – used to picture *Gladiator*-style blokes lifting massive weights and think it was basically about brute strength. But it's about so much more than that. Our muscles are hugely protective, keep our bodies ticking over in perfect balance and are, ultimately, life-extending.

I am now focusing on building and looking after my muscle strength, in a way that I simply wasn't a few years ago. In this chapter, I'm going to share with you the reasons *why* muscles are incredible, the risks we're exposing ourselves to if we neglect them, busting the sexist myths that have put women off so far, and how we can all build muscle strength to futureproof ourselves and ensure a healthy, independent life.

SO, WHAT ACTUALLY *ARE* MUSCLES?

The reason why our muscles are an organ is because of their size and function. They have all sorts of jobs to do in our body – far too many for us to detail here, otherwise it'll end up like a biology lesson! But I will give you the important overview: our muscles are an endocrine (hormonal) organ, helping all our other organs regulate loads of body functions by communicating with them – it's like they are listening and talking to the rest of our body. There are three types of muscle tissue – skeletal, cardiac and smooth – and they all have different roles.[1]

- **Cardiac**: this is the stuff that's around our heart and keeps our blood pumping. Cardiac muscle tissue works *involuntarily*, which means we don't control it; it contracts and relaxes without any intervention from us. So we can leave that one here!
- **Smooth**: these muscle fibres are in the walls of our visceral organs, like the liver, bladder and intestines. Again, they are involuntary muscles and work independently.
- **Skeletal**: This is the one we're going to focus on. Skeletal muscle is sometimes referred to as the 'exoskeleton' as it's joined to our bones, so it keeps our skeleton in place and enables us to move – without it, we would be a heap of clattering bones! It makes up around 40 per cent of our entire body weight and is in *voluntary* control – meaning we control its movement. It responds to messages from our nervous system, our complex network of cells and fibres throughout the body.

A great way to explain why skeletal muscle is so important is that it's the 'internal engine that drives all systems'. I've borrowed this from a brilliant doctor called Dr Gabrielle Lyon, who founded a movement called Muscle-Centric Medicine and has written a fabulous book called *Forever Strong* (another one for your bedside table). She is utterly passionate about improving muscle health as a vital tool for longevity, as am I! We need to flip our received wisdom about muscles and instead see them as a suit of armour, protecting us and futureproofing us.

BUT AREN'T MUSCLES JUST ABOUT STRENGTH?

This used to be me – I honestly used to believe that the only benefit of building muscles was that you'd be able to bench some impressive weights in the gym. That it was all about the *physical health* benefits. But what I've been staggered to discover in recent times is the multitude of ways that muscle mass impacts our longevity. And the reason for this is its role in our **metabolic health.**

In the last chapter, we talked about a major metabolic problem called *insulin resistance,* and how being inflamed led to a sluggish metabolism, where our bodies can't use our energy stores effectively. As we've already seen, a crappy metabolic function is behind so many life-limiting diseases. What's amazing, though, is how important quality muscles are for powering a better metabolic function, and therefore a longer healthspan.

Improved muscle mass means you change how your body processes food and energy. This is because better muscle mass increases our density of muscle *mitochondria* – the tiny units in our cell walls that produce energy from the food we eat. Basically, we work more effectively. And there are loads of additional benefits from better muscular metabolic health, too. For example:

It stabilises our blood sugar without insulin

Our muscles perform this amazing job by releasing amino acids (the building blocks for proteins) which synthesise our glucose levels in the liver. They do this *without* the need for insulin, by taking the glucose first and converting it to glycogen to restore our energy levels.

Now, this is very handy, because it therefore saves our insulin levels from going too high or too low, and reduces our risk of developing type 2 diabetes (and sadly, we become far more insulin resistant as we get older, so this becomes more of an issue). Even if we are already dealing with diabetes, this also shows us just how lifting weights and doing squats will improve our blood-sugar regulation much more than all this 'just go for a gentle walk' nonsense ... We need things like walking lunges and squats to power our muscles and insulin balance (and more on this later!).

It powers our immune system

Inflammation is the culprit behind so many diseases, which we explored in depth in the last chapter. Brilliantly, having strong skeletal muscles also boosts our immunity and reduces inflammation by releasing *myokines* when we work out. Myokines are cytokines – small peptide proteins – released by muscles and are absorbed into the bloodstream. (You may remember that there are both pro- and anti-inflammatory cytokines – the *anti*-inflammatory sorts are the ones we want!)

These peptides send powerful signals throughout our body that reduce inflammation and fight off disease.[2] This is why muscle-building exercises have been shown not only to suppress the growth of tumours, but improve the outcomes of those with cancer,[3] showing just how super, super-important they are for our long-term health.

It burns fat, even at rest

By increasing our metabolic function, lean muscle mass helps us burn more energy more quickly – not only during exercise, but after it too.[4] Being muscular means your body is more capable of burning through body-fat-inducing ingredients like pasta and breads. These carby foods convert to glucose, which, as we know, can cause weight gain if consumed and stored excessively. This is fabulous news for us people who can't give up carbohydrates – myself included – so if we want to enjoy them, we have to build muscle.

It boosts our brain health

Muscle-building is good for the whole of our nervous system because it literally fires everything up. It creates an increase in blood flow, so we have more oxygen and nutrients flooding our cells all over the body and, fabulously, it lights up a particular part of the brain that is only switched on from strength training! A scientist called Eric Kandel even won the Nobel Prize by discovering that muscle-building (load-bearing) exercises stimulate the release of a hormone called *osteocalcin*. This travels to the brain and enhances our neural health and improves memory, keeping us sharp.[5]

As well as these metabolic advantages, the physical benefits are phenomenal, too. Not only will we get stronger, and more energised, but we'll strengthen our bones too, reducing our pain risk from osteoarthritis in later life, which is especially vital for women (I've written more on this later on; but the contraction and release in muscle-building exercise causes bones to feel pressure. This, in turn, builds bone density and stability and means we're less likely to suffer from fractures. Ta-da!)

WHY MUSCLE STRENGTH IS IMPORTANT FOR LONGEVITY

I hope this has given you some new insights into why muscles matter so much. They are what we all need to prioritise – not only for staving off disease and other hallmarks of ageing, but to enjoy all the benefits of good health, too. 'The more skeletal muscle mass an individual has, the greater your survivability,' Dr Gabrielle says. Truly, we ignore our muscles at our own peril!

So, not only do I want to be more muscular because it makes my immune system stronger, my bones denser, my brain sharper, it also means I can eat sourdough, potatoes and the odd pizza – all the things I still love. (I won't be having veg oils, though ... no solution for that stuff.) The more I dive into it, the more I am staggered not only by how vital they are, but how little we have been focusing on muscles. After all, when was the last time your doctor told you to build muscle to preserve and improve your health? Scientist and endurance expert Dr Andy Galpin agrees, saying on *The Huberman Lab* that 'one of the major disservices that has been done ... is convincing people that things like strength training are only for athletes or for growing bigger and building muscles – this leads to a lot of false assumptions and poor actions'.

No matter – we can change this. We can enjoy all the benefits of better blood glucose, better stability, better bone strength, better mood, and reduce our risk of disease by focusing on building muscle strength. And this is extra vital as we get older.

SARCOPENIA AND MUSCLE WASTAGE

One of the hallmarks of ageing is our physical strength diminishing. Sorry to drop this on you, but our natural muscle mass peaks when we're about thirty and then begins to deplete from then on. The actual rates will naturally vary between individuals, but on average we lose about 1 per cent of our muscle size and around 2 per cent of our muscle strength *per year* from the age of forty. After we hit seventy, this then accelerates to about 15 per cent per decade!

This process of muscle wastage and reduced muscle mass is called *sarcopenia,* and it can have horrendous consequences – longevity expert Dr Peter Attia says in his book *Outlive*: 'continued muscle loss and inactivity literally puts our lives at risk'. So the older we get, the *more* we need to build muscle mass, not only for the incredible benefits we've seen, but to stave off this natural sarcopenic process. If we do not do any muscle-building exercises and sit around eating complete rubbish, then sarcopenia will result in us losing muscle mass, developing weaker bones, stiffer joints and poor balance – all of which lead to more falls.

WHY FALLING CAN BE FATAL

How many times have you heard the older people in your life talk about 'having a fall'? We might sometimes roll our eyes at our ageing parents or grandparents fretting about this – and sidebar, at what age does 'falling over' become 'having a fall?' There seems to be an official changeover date in the language at some point! But to be fair, it is a worrying business when you get older. The stats bear this out, and in all sorts of shocking ways.

Here are a few. Falls are *by far* the leading cause of injury-related death in the over-sixty-fives in both the US[6] and the UK.[7] Injuries from falls cost the NHS more than £2bn a year.[8] Hip fractures are one of the most common injuries sustained in falling, and one in three people with a hip fracture die within the year.[9] This isn't just because of the injury itself, but from the consequences of being bedbound and losing even more muscle mass, plus diminished immunity from all the medications, etc., etc. Discovering that, for me, was a real oh-my-God moment. And no wonder people fear falls – Age UK found that millions of older people said it was top of their list of concerns.[10] They can literally happen at any moment.

Just recently, a friend of mine saw an elderly woman simply step off the bus and immediately slam down on to the pavement, seriously injuring herself. I bet every single one of you reading has either seen an old person fall or had someone in their family suffer badly after falling. It is so common. For this reason, it's absolutely vital that we stay steady on our feet and that means building muscle in our core and our legs.

IT'S NEVER TOO LATE TO START!

This all sounds very doom-and-gloomy, but hurray hurray, it is completely possible to move out of a sarcopenic state and prevent our future from being one of those grim stats. People with more muscle mass fall less because they have increased core, back and limb strength, as well as better co-ordination and quicker responses. They are not only more stable but can catch themselves before they fall, and if a fall does happen, they recover more quickly from injury. Overall, *they live longer.*

We can all build this protective, life-extending muscle mass through exercising and, specifically, through *resistance training.* It is literally the number one way to build quality muscle mass that we have at our disposal, and we can introduce it at any age. Truly!

It doesn't matter if you're in your sixties, seventies or even beyond; *everyone* should do strength training. Interestingly, stats show that it really is never too late to see amazing results. Even at the age of ninety-plus (yes, ninety!), it's been demonstrated that you can improve your muscle strength by over 120 per cent in a few weeks.[11] That sounds unbelievable, but it is true – there really is no such thing as leaving it 'too late'. I'm not saying you should *wait* until you're that old, far from it, but it's good news to know that your muscles are this quick to respond to a bit of love and attention.

If you're feeling resistance to the whole idea of resistance training – and you're not alone in this, let me assure you – let me explain why going for a stroll around the park won't suffice.

WHY JUST DOING CARDIO ISN'T ENOUGH

It's long been understood just how important cardio exercise is for longevity and I am not here to tell you to stop doing your Zumba, or running, or HIIT training if you're already doing it. Keep going! Literally, jog on! But we cannot rely on cardio alone to futureproof us: Dr Gabrielle puts it brilliantly, explaining that cardio doesn't 'supply sufficient fuel to power muscle growth'. If we only focus on cardio-based exercising, we'll end up losing *both* fat and muscle mass over time, which is not what we want! So, we have to introduce weight-bearing training into our routines.

Every single expert out there with a specialism in longevity and healthspan will tell you that resistance training to build muscle is essential to combat this neuromuscular ageing. It is the only way to get bodily younger. This is a million miles away from some of the more out-there biohacking protocols that cost a fortune – building muscle mass is something we can all do, and very affordably.

We need to do it now, not wait until we've injured ourselves and need to rebuild strength – that will be so much harder. We want to futureproof ourselves against this. Dr Peter Attia calls this approach 'prehab' – getting ahead of the catastrophe, rather than responding to it. I'm all for that!

WHY DOES RESISTANCE TRAINING BUILD MUSCLE MASS?

'Resistance training' means any exercise that builds strength by causing muscles to contract against an external force (a 'resistance'). The resistance could come in the form of dumbbells, kettlebells, weight machines, stretchy exercise bands, medicine balls, or even your own body weight – just think of planks. (And just so you know, the terms 'strength training', 'resistance training' and 'muscle training' are often used interchangeably – they all mean basically the same thing.) Any exercise you do where you are pushing against an external force is resistance training. So, it includes things like lifting weights – either free weights or on a weights machine; squats and lunges;

doing sit-ups; and chin-ups, which happens to be my own personal goal.

The reason resistance training is so brilliant at building muscle mass is because it damages the muscle fibres, which are long and thin, a bit like a ponytail. This sounds counter-intuitive – after all, if they're damaged, aren't they screwed? Ah, but no – they have tons of fibres, which break and repair, getting stronger and stronger the more we work out and push ourselves.

This is because resistance training activates a molecule called mTOR (which stands for mammalian target of rapamycin – yep, *I know* this sounds like a terrible fantasy novel), which regulates how we synthesise protein. Our amazing bodies rely on the mTOR signalling to build muscle, so over time, with more mTOR, our muscles get stronger and more defined.[12]

What's more, this process also encourages autophagy, which we covered in the previous chapter on inflammation – but without fasting! The most important thing we need to know, though, is that through resistance training, not only will we build muscle, but we'll also repair damaged cells and our hair, skin, nails and even gut. There is an abundance of amazing benefits to be had.

HOW I GOT STARTED BUILDING MUSCLE MASS

Full disclosure here: I was late to the muscle-building party. I should have focused on this in my twenties, but let's be honest, I wasn't making many healthy choices back then! But even when I began exercising properly in my thirties, it was completely natural for me to lean towards running. It suits my personality in so many ways. I love listening to music, getting into my own personal rhythm, and being on my own – I can be a bit of a lone wolf! – so running is my default setting as it ticks all those boxes. I found it very hard to prioritise working on my muscles because I simply did not get anywhere near the same enjoyment from doing weights. You can't get distracted because you've got to think more about what you're doing and count reps – and admin is not my forte, to put it mildly . . .

So, a few years ago, to get me going properly, I started working with a personal trainer, Charlie. He was a proper lad, no bullshit, and really helped me get motivated – as well as declutter all the other noise going on in my brain that would have prevented me from properly working out. I must be honest, though. When I first came to him, I had a lot of existing baggage around the idea of building muscle and was worried about getting 'too' muscly. Like many girls and women, I had been indoctrinated to fear it as something unfeminine and unattractive (and I will go into why this is such self-harming crap shortly!). So, when he proposed all these muscle-building exercises, my response was 'OK, but I don't want to bulk up, I just want to lose weight.'

He laughed his head off. 'There's not a cat's chance in hell you're going to get bigger,' he told me. 'You're not going to be benching anywhere near enough. It's just not going to happen.' It was one of the biggest, and best, reality checks I've ever had. He was pissing himself at my bonkers notion that I would pick up a few weights and immediately look like a bodybuilder. I loved that, because it made me realise how crazy that thinking was.

The simple fact is that it's very, very difficult for women to bulk up. You cannot do it without serious amounts of nuanced work and probably a lot of steroids, too. Of course, we're not going to go anywhere *near* this! And like Charlie made me realise, it will not just 'happen' the second we start resistance training. The more I think about it, the more I realise how ridiculous it was. I mean, come on, who was I kidding?!

GETTING STRONGER, NOT BIGGER

So, one of the first big steps women should take is unhooking this association between building muscle and bulking up. It's a common misconception to link the two together and is usually the number one reason that women don't use weights. However, it is not surprising most women think like this. After all, for decades, images of pumped-up guys and a narrative that equates having huge muscles with hyper-masculinity have been around us all – affecting both women's and men's perception of muscle-building. But women just do not need to worry about bulking up, unless there is a focus on becoming an Olympic-level boxer or entering a bodybuilding competition, which I assume 99.9 per cent are *not* intending to do.

It is entirely possible to get stronger and leaner *without* building volume. Some of the strongest people in the world are not 'big': they're yogis, gymnasts, ballet dancers, Pilates experts. You only have to spend a few minutes on the internet watching videos of people balancing on one arm, or gymnasts performing incredible moves, or the gravity-defying feats in a ballet performance to realise that **super-strong does not equal super-size**. These lean and stable people can lift and hold their own body weight, do pull-ups, jump to huge heights – and literally everything they do is powered by their majorly strong muscles!

To be honest, it makes me rage when I think about how much women have been taught to fear building muscle. Because as

I've found out, women need to futureproof muscle strength just as much as men – and in some ways, more. It is literally the key to independence and a pain-free life.

FIGHTING THE 'BLOKEY' STEREOTYPE

If you're about my age, you probably remember the utter media frenzy that kicked off a few years ago when Madonna showed off her muscly arms. People were completely grossed out by it, and the criticism that was levelled at her was *insane* – she was called things like 'manly' and 'blokey', amongst the milder insults. Fortunately, nowadays I don't think that level of sexist condemnation would pass muster – we wouldn't insult somebody for looking different. We've moved on a bit in how we treat people's different shapes, and it's socially unacceptable to body-shame. If someone wrote that now, they would probably be immediately cancelled!

However, this doesn't mean women no longer have to deal with the bullshit stereotypes of what is 'sexy' or 'attractive'. Women are still under massive pressure from society – in everything from social media to advertising, to our mates – to look a certain way. And there has definitely been a dominant social narrative on losing weight above all else. Many women are simply scared of putting muscle on top of the body fat they already have because there's a fear it'll end up in getting wider. I used to think like that, too. But not only will women *not* get any bigger, we will actually shrink our body fat by getting more muscular. We will be leaner, stronger and burn excess fuel even when we're at rest. We will not be 'over-masculine'. Sod that! We will be strong and resilient.

WHY STRONG MUSCLES = STRONG BONES = STRONG FUTURE

There are so many reasons why it's extra, extra-important for women to preserve and maintain muscle health. Firstly, because they are more likely to deal with bone-density health issues as they age. Osteoporosis, where bones become more fragile, and bone pain with osteoarthritis are a huge problem for millions of women after the menopause. It's a complex issue, but research now shows that hormonal birth control can have an adverse effect on bone health. Taking the contraceptive pill or having the 'depo' DMPA injection, especially during adolescence, results in lower bone-mineral density (BMD) levels.[13] In essence, this means women have an even higher risk of developing bone problems later in life!

This sounds terrifying, because many women – me included – took the pill when we were teenagers, chucking it down our throats without a second thought and thinking we looked dead cool. (Health authorities in the States have even warned teens against having the depo injection specifically because of this issue.)[14] Argh, I can hear many of you cry, it's too late for me! However, there are things to do – not least by firstly making sure we encourage any of our daughters and sons or friends to educate themselves about the potential outcomes of hormonal birth control. Secondly, all of us can start building muscle to futureproof ourselves. The good news is it's been clearly proven that strength training not only increases muscle mass, but also increases bone density.[15] Through this, we can all begin to mitigate the negative effects that reduced bone density might have on our future.

You might think I'm exaggerating the risks, but having strong bones is *such* a big deal for women. With osteoporosis, we are more likely to live a life in pain, or with reduced mobility and broken bones. Stats show that up to 60 per cent of people who break their hip never regain full independence.[16] None of us want this! And women have to be extra vigilant, especially because they live longer than men. Nobody wants to end up living in a dreaded old-age purgatory where we've lost all our dignity. But by ignoring our muscle health, we are setting ourselves up for a flimsy future.

One of my favourite pieces of new technology which is going to massively support women and men in building bone density is the bioDensity machine.[17] The way it works is it allows you to perform high-impact exercises without the usual risks associated with heavy lifting or jumping. The machine puts your body into the optimal position to cope with a heavy load, and only asks you to exert your full energy for five seconds per movement (pushing against weight using your arms and legs). This makes it perfect for anyone who is new to resistance training or in their later years. Studies have shown that through weekly sessions, this machine can improve bone density to combat osteoporosis and osteopenia. Sounds like minimal effort for maximum results!

This machine is now available in a number of locations around the world and conveniently at a clinic run by Gary Rhodes not too far from me in the north of England. Gary was motivated to get into the field when his much-loved grandmother began suffering with osteoporosis. His clinic, DexaStrong, offers bone-density therapy, using the bioDensity machine, as well as bio-density scanning using the Dexa machine. I got the opportunity to have one of these scans and it showed me that I probably do need to do a little less running and a little more gym work. My bones look pretty good, but are on the lower side of normal, and since I am on a journey to optimising my bone health, I am going to commit to spending more time lifting weights and using the bioDensity machine when I can. I am also going to add supplements that have been proven to aid bone density, such as calcium hydroxyapatite, up my vitamin D3 (through supplementation teamed with magnesium and MK-7 and daily sunlight exposure) and explore all the amazing minerals that can help too. I am particularly intrigued by boron, phosphorus and zinc. Not only will I be adding all this in, I'll also be watching my stress and sugar intake as these can have awful impacts on bone density.

If you can't get to a bioDensity machine, I found out through talking to dentist Dr Usman Riaz, Renovo Dental, that it is possible to detect osteoporosis with a routine dental X-ray.[18] By looking at age, weight and hormone levels alongside it, Dr Usman's clinic can provide a risk score for possible development of osteoporosis in the future. This is an evolving science and not used diagnostically in the same way we use a DEXA scan, but he has been conducting this screening service at Renovo dental for a year and is so excited by the potential of this kind of preventative approach.

So, to all women, I say forget all the crap we've been fed about building muscles being unsexy and masculine. It's bollocks! Looking after muscles is not a lads' thing, it's an *everyone* thing. We all need decent strength to protect us, keep us alive and thriving. Knowing what we know now, let's not use fear of bulking up as an excuse against muscle-building. That 'oh, but I don't want to get any bigger' argument just doesn't hold up to scrutiny, and overall only does *you* a huge disservice, not anyone else.

We are going to flip all this nonsense on its head and instead of setting ourselves up for vulnerability, we will lay the foundations for resilience. (I know I've already talked about resilience, but you're just going to have to cope with me banging on about it throughout this book!) By focusing on muscles, we'll have all increased our safety, our strength and our mental health.

THE POTENTIAL POWER OF CALCIUM HYDROXYAPATITE

I first learned about calcium hydroxyapatite from my brilliant dentist Dr Usman Riaz. Dr Usman calls it the 'super mineral' because, he told me, 'your body can use it to repair itself'.

He went on to explain that calcium hydroxyapatite 'is a naturally occurring form of the mineral calcium apatite – calcium, phosphorus and oxygen – that grows in hexagonal crystals. It makes up most of the human bone structure, builds tooth enamel and collects in tiny amounts in part of the brain.'

We have always known about the great regenerative properties of hydroxyapatite. So why the fuss? Only now, after recent breakthroughs in nanotechnology, is it possible to make this highly sought after substance in a lab setting for medical uses – this is a real game changer. This lab-created substance is called hydroxyapatite. Hydroxyapatite is a rare material, in that it is a 'bioactive material', so it is one of the few lab-made materials that will help bones and teeth grow!

The mineral is already present in our bones and teeth but can also be used by medical professionals when repairing bone breaks or loss. Dr Usman is a big fan of hydroxyapatite toothpaste instead of fluoride toothpaste as he says 'it offers the same remineralising benefits as fluoride without the toxicity risks'. At this point, studies are limited, but with more research to come, he says 'the regenerative potential of this mineral is remarkable.'

HOW TO BUILD MUSCLE AND FUTUREPROOF YOURSELF

Reasons to be cheerful

The good news right here, right now, about muscle-building is that *you will see quick gains.* I promise you! Unlike fat or weight loss, which takes a very long time to kick in, once you start exercising to build muscle mass, you will see noticeable physical changes in your body in less than six weeks, often in as little as a fortnight (and as long as you're committed). No matter what your current one-rep max is (your one-rep max is the absolute maximum weight you can lift once), *you will improve it*, in a way that is meaningful to you. All the problem areas you might have, like your abdominals, weak glutes or bingo wings, we can get them stronger and leaner.

What's more, you'll not only look better on the outside, with a more defined shape, you'll feel so much better on the inside as well. Your brain will be sharper, you'll have improved cognition and better moods. You'll feel stronger and more energised, more confident and secure in yourself. This should be a powerful motivator even if you don't love exercise right now. There really are only wins to be had here.

The first thing you should do is . . .

The first piece of advice I'm going to give you is to join a gym, if you haven't done so already. Now, before you throw this book down in a rage and think, *Forget it, there's no way I'm doing that, are you nuts?* Hold on! Hear me out! The reason I say this is because I don't want to patronise you by claiming that lifting up a couple of tins of beans in your kitchen while waiting for the kettle to boil will give you the same results as lifting proper weights in a gym. It won't; it's just not possible. This kind of 'advice' is pointless and it's been done to death. I've lost track of the times I've read this sort of nonsense, and I bet you have too.

There are exercises you can do at home – of course there are – and if joining a gym is completely unavailable to you, I will outline some alternative options later in this chapter. But I will say that there is no better place to build muscle strength and resilience than at the gym. There just isn't. This might sound a bit brutal, but I don't see the point in mollycoddling you, or conning you that results will miraculously appear without real effort. I've been there, looking for easy fixes, and I know that they don't work. Instead, let's be honest with ourselves about what we really need to do, and not be wet wipes!

FLIPPING THE THINKING: WHY 'BUT I CAN'T' DOESN'T HOLD UP!

I've heard every weird and wonderful excuse possible why people 'can't' join a gym – even my mate Becky claims she doesn't want to go because she doesn't like 'the smell'!

Honestly. But in most cases, I can give you loads of reasons why you can and should flip this resistance on its head. Below are some of the most common things I hear and how I can persuade you otherwise! (And just to be clear: I used to fall back on some of these excuses myself, so there's no judgement if this is you right now . . .)

'I can't fit it in'

Unless you have literally every minute of every hour of every day already accounted for, I'll challenge you on this! Everyone working out in any gym across the UK right now has *other* stuff to do. They've all got families, jobs, responsibilities, lists of boring stuff they've got to pick up from Tesco – it's not as if they can only go because they have no demands on their time. What they're doing that's different is fitting it in. Finding the space in their day to prioritise their health. Just getting on with it.

If it was true that everyone was far 'too busy' to work out, then gyms would go out of business because nobody would be in them. Netflix wouldn't be worth around $250 billion because everyone would be 'too busy' to watch it. Stats wouldn't show that us Brits watch an average of more than two hours of TV per day[19] (and I count myself in this group of telly addicts!). You get my point. We can always fit in the stuff we *want* to fit in.

I know I'm lucky that I can set my own schedule, and not everyone can. I'm able to work out in the morning after the kids' drop-off and get into my office a bit later on. Even if I wasn't self-employed, though, I would still do it before I went to work because I'm a morning person. Getting up at 5 a.m. I can do, but staying up past 9 p.m.?

Nope, that wouldn't work for me! But it might be perfect for you. The point is, you've got to put yourself first and work out how you can make room for the gym in your life, in a way that suits you best. If you've got kids, they will see this and try to emulate you. If you start to feel guilty, spin it: they are learning self-care from you.

'I can work out just as well at home'

The truth of the matter is, you won't push yourself properly at home. You might be the most motivated person on earth, but you can't do a superset, you can't lift real weights if all you've got are some Aldi dumbbells. Going to the gym gives you access to incredible stuff that costs thousands of pounds and will target specific areas to build muscle.

I understand if you've been working out at home because you feel self-conscious in front of other people. But let me reassure you: no one gives a shit what you look like in a gym. Loads of people of all shapes, sizes and ages go to my local gym, people with disabilities, they're all in there, getting on with it. I promise, nobody is there to laugh at or mock you, because everyone knows what it's like to start from day one. They might acknowledge you with a nod, but everyone is just super-focused on doing their own stuff.

'I can't afford it!'

Long gone are the days where gyms were only for the wealthy – in the last few years there has been a real explosion of budget-style gyms, where pools and saunas have been ditched (which were the extras that really bumped up the membership price). There is *so* much cost variety out there, depending on the gym and where you live. However, there are bargains to be had, especially when you sign up somewhere new.

We all have loads of expenses in our lives, and gyms can really feel like a 'nice to have' rather than an essential. But for the cost of a couple of Starbucks sugar bombs a week – have you *seen* the prices in coffee shops, recently? – you can take up a gym membership that will bring you untold benefits instead. If you can make some budget adjustments, swap or move your spending around from one pot to a gym pot, do it.

'I don't like gyms'

Not all gyms are the same! You can find the place that's right for you. I used to care about the coolest gyms where everyone was in Sweaty Betty, and there are gyms that have great lighting and make you look fabulous if that's what you need. Ask to have a look around your local gyms to get an idea of what's out there – you don't need to join up to a membership just to pop your head in. I love lads' gyms now because I feel safe there, and I know what I'm doing. But I get so much more out of the gym than just the kit and the right weights – I get a sense of community.

We all remember the horrible times during Covid, where we were isolated, depressed and stuck in our homes. Let's not isolate ourselves all over again by hiding away when we work out. At a gym, you soon make friends with the receptionist, recognise the PT who took your baseline info, chat about the weather with a couple of regulars.

You build a little neighbourhood of people; you feel part of something that is way more than just a room full of weights. I've talked a lot before about how we are all part of a human tribe, and we need each other. So going to the gym is more than the physical benefits – it really boosts our mental and emotional wellbeing by connecting us with a community.

'None of my friends go to the gym!'

If your mates don't want to come with you, and they want to stay at home drinking Prosexy and watching Netflix, or going to the pub, that's fine. Keep the friends you have, especially if they are good, loyal mates, but you can always find another tribe at the gym. In any case, a lot of us find we develop different lifestyles from our old friends over the years.

This is the situation I have in my own life – I'm the only one who doesn't drink any more out of my school mates. They still go out and get absolutely bladdered and I'm there for the stories and the chat afterwards, but I have different tribes now, too, including my gym crowd and the online biohacking community. I have tried to persuade my school mates to come to the gym, but my best mate has said, more than once, 'Don't be so fucking ridiculous!' She just doesn't want to, and I have to accept that. So, you *can* be the first in your group to go to the gym, you can get over your fear and find a new tribe. You be the pioneer.

'Gyms are too blokey'

Right (cracks knuckles), this is a big one. Gyms can sometimes feel as if they are such a macho space, and lots of women can feel social anxiety about going into them for this reason. I get this. I think it's especially tricky to consider gyms if you've never been in one before and all you've heard is lads bragging loudly about what they're lifting! (I remember when I was young and going out in Wigan at night with my friend Harvey – we would piss ourselves at all the gym bros at the bars with their tight T-shirts, perfect gelled hair and fake tan asking each other, 'What you benching?' It was *hilarious*.) I now say, 'What's your one-rep max?' to my lads, who find me beyond annoying.

My sons are now moving into their 'benching' phase and are obsessed with getting ripped. It's the reason what was *supposed* to be my lovely telly room at home now looks absolutely horrible, with weights, crash pads and a bloody mirror leaning up against a wall. They are in there constantly, pratting around, lifting weights. I'll have to wait a few years for my own TV room it seems.

But knowing what I know about muscles, I'm happy to let them make absolute tools of themselves wittering on in gym jargon, because I know the long-term mental and physical health benefits are a million times better than them going out and getting shitfaced. The sad thing is, we just don't see teen girls flocking to the gym in the same way, do we? There doesn't seem to be the social pressure for them to build muscle with their mates. And as we've seen from all the data, girls more than anyone should be learning how to weight-train from their teens; not in a competitive way, but in a protective way.

The culture might currently skew in favour of boys being utter benchers, but we can all change this. Everyone can start role-modelling to the younger generation by getting down the gym and demonstrating that it's a space for all of us.

Four ways to get motivated for the gym

If we're going to make muscle-building fitness a long-term part of our life, rather than something we drop after the novelty wears off, we need to make the whole process as motivating as possible. Here are some ways to do it that really work for me and give me more intention to work out.

1. Rev yourself up with music

As those of you who've read my last book, *Hack Your Hormones,* will know, we are wired to seek out our pleasure receptors as much as possible, through our dopamine response. It's all too easy to get a dopamine hit from doughnuts or wine, but we can turn the gym into a pleasurable, positive source of it instead.

We can do this first by making the build-up really stimulating. Put a feel-good playlist together ahead of time, and blast that out in the car, or through your headphones on the bus or your walk to the gym, to get yourself revved up. When you're there, turn off your alerts and put your phone on silent so you don't get distracted by messages from friends, work or annoying apps. (Having said that, I have been known to do my emails while incline walking on the treadmill!) But throughout your session, keep those tunes going. By soundtracking our gym experience with uplifting music, we'll access our pleasure receptors and that dopamine response more quickly, which will encourage us to push a lot harder.

How music gets me motivated

I use music in all sorts of ways to power me in my workouts, whether that's at the gym, outside or at home. I've learned that different sorts of tunes are brilliant for getting me going in different ways – autonomically, your body adapts to the rhythm of the music, so higher-intensity music tends to lead to higher-intensity effort. Something mundane, or even too emotional, just won't work the same way. Here's how music works for me, so have a play around to see which tunes fire you up and make you feel good for different workouts.

- *For a slow run on a summer's day:* easy-listening 80s soul music like Luther Vandross – 'Give Me the Night'
- *When I'm rucking on an incline walk:* 70s disco is perfect (and more on rucking later). Sister Sledge – 'Lost in Music'
- *A full-on workout:* I need to access that euphoric recall I got from going into a club when I was young, so I go back to 1996 and get some banging house tunes on from that era
- *To motivate me when I can't be bothered:* soundtracks to 80s movies like *Back to the Future* and *Dirty Dancing* are really nostalgic for me and take me right back to the junior disco!

I love hearing what gets people moving – the more cringe the better I say!

2. Wear kit that gives you confidence

By this, I don't mean spending £££ on the most expensive gym kit going (although if this is what works for you, knock yourself out!). What I mean is the workout kit that means you're not worrying about what you look like – the stuff that is comfortable, that keeps your body protected and secure.

For example, if I have runners' shorts on, I always wear leggings underneath them, just because that makes me feel more confident that my arse isn't going to be hanging out. And for women, if you're on your period, just wear all-black stuff so you're not worried about leaks. (Actually, you may as well wear black all the time, because as we know, our periods can and do sometimes come out of nowhere. A friend of mine came on when she was about to run a half-marathon and spent the whole thirteen miles fretting that she was going to bleed through her light-blue running shorts. Nightmare.)

We're starting to hear more about the risk of forever plastics in our workout clothes entering our bloodstream more easily while we're sweating in them during exercise. Now, if you've got all the money in the world and want to source kit that is plastic free, go for it. However, my approach is that it is better to make it to the gym in whatever kit you find comfortable and affordable, take it off as soon as you get home, and don't overthink it. Getting to the gym in whatever clothes you've got to hand is a net positive in my book. There are other ways we can deal with inflammation from the toxins in our environment. Bloody hell, we've got enough to worry about without panicking about the material our kit is made of!

Whatever your worry, save yourself the mental paranoia and the hassle, and get your hands on some kit that means you can focus on the workout rather than what you look like.

3. Document your progress

This is notepad time! As I've explained, you are going to see major gains once you start strength training – gains are not just for twenty-two-year-old lads in JD Sports! So, what you need to do is document where you're at, so you can log how much you improve.

It doesn't need to be essay-length stuff; at the end of each session, jot down the date and your personal numbers. This could include your one-rep max for lifting weights, the number of push-ups you managed, how long you held a wall squat for – really, *whatever* you are doing, log it. Keep a special gym notepad in your kit bag so you've always got it to hand and make a point of looking back at how far you've come every few weeks. You will be astonished and super-motivated to see how much you progress.

4. Share it with friends

There are different ways your friends can help power you forward on your strength-building journey. One way is by having a gym buddy with you to spur you on (as long as you don't end up just chatting with them for ages, which I have done plenty of times!). You can then return the favour and it'll be a huge stimulus for both of you to work stronger.

Even if you don't have a friend that can join you, get your mates involved by sharing what you're doing. Whether that's on social media, or on a WhatsApp group, make them a part of it. Not only will their encouragement help you (and if they're good mates, they should be encouraging rather than not), but you never know, you might just suddenly inspire somebody else. You should also be honest with your mates if you're losing the momentum or urge to go. Hopefully they'll call you out and give you the reminder you need that you have never regretted a workout.

Listen, *whatever* gets you through the door of the gym, do it. All these suggestions might seem like little things, but they're geared towards achieving an important goal – to help you build healthy habits. You need to feel at home in the gym. That it's *your* special place where you are safeguarding your future. We are all a work in progress; none of us are the finished product, but we can make these positive changes. All it takes is literally one day out of your life to shift its trajectory – and we *can* do it.

My favourite unusual muscle-building exercises to do in the gym

I'd always recommend getting some expert advice from your gym's PTs first, especially when it comes to using the equipment effectively and safely. Of course, it would be impossible (and make this book very, very long) to list everything you *could* do to focus on muscle strength when you're down the gym. But here are a few of my favourite muscle-strengthening exercises that are brilliant and might not be the most obvious ones . . .

One-leg bench presses
I spoke to a gym instructor at a longevity clinic recently and he advised me to bench-press using one leg at a time, rather than both at once. The reason for this is that very rarely do we push using equal energy on both legs! We end up using one leg more and so the other side doesn't get strong. To get around this, we should adjust our workout so we bench-press with one leg, then the other; this is a great little hack to ensure muscle-building doesn't end up uneven!

3D weight training

One brilliant piece of biohackery to make your gym workout more effective is to train in three dimensions, which means across all three planes of movement – sagittal, frontal and transverse. Here's a quick summary to try and make it less confusing!

- Sagittal plane: forwards/backwards/up/down movements, e.g. lunges
- Frontal plane: sideways movements, e.g. side planks
- Transverse plane: rotating/parallel movements e.g. push-ups[20]

This might sound confusing, but here's an example. Say you are doing bicep curls with a light dumbbell. Instead of just lifting them up and down from your elbow, which is moving through only one plane (sagittal), you could rotate your arms too and activate more muscles. Chat with the gym staff on how to introduce 3D training into your workout.

Go down as well as up

We've all heard a million times about how important it is to walk up hills, to take the steps instead of the escalator, all of that, haven't we? And it is – but what doesn't get discussed enough is just how important our 'step-down' strength is. As we age, this lack of steadiness with weak ankles is what causes us to fall more, so being able to step on and off a kerb safely and strongly is vital. And without lateral ankle strength, we can't build muscle in the rest of our body effectively.[21]

So, we need to set our treadmill to a 'decline' setting, not just an incline. Walking downwards on the treadmill will build muscle strength and flexibility in our ankles, as well as our quadriceps (the front part of our thighs).[22] Mix up your treadmill work so that it incorporates this ankle flexor strength-building, too.

Bring back the Power Plate

Available on eBay or in some gyms, the Power Plate helps to strengthen and build muscle even faster. Vibration therapy has also been shown to help reduce stress as it activates the parasympathetic branch of your central nervous system.

If you really, really, REALLY can't join a gym

By now I've done the best I can to convince you to give gyms a go, but I understand that this simply might be completely unavailable to you. You might have iron-clad reasons why you can't, such as childcare issues (although many gyms have a crèche now, so check your local ones out), an impossible schedule, or you live somewhere that makes going to the gym completely out of reach. Or it could be something else – that's fine. So if you've been yelling at me these last few pages, *but I really, really CAN'T join a gym for frig's sake,* I hear you! There are plenty of things you can do from home, with or without specialist kit. And the first thing you need to get sorted is an absolutely banging playlist.

To do from home: the three-track dopamine muscle workout

Regardless of whether you are going to a gym or not, or if you haven't exercised in ages, you need to boost your dopamine. This is mind-over-matter stuff. We want to hack into the feel-good hormones to get you motivated and set the tone for making it as enjoyable as possible. So, ahead of time, sort out that playlist and make it amazing. Get outside in the morning, get your light exposure, get your coffee or matcha tea or cacao – whatever it is that gives you an *oomph*. I will often take WillPowders Brain Powder; it's got nootropics in which boost mental and physical motivation via the dopamine-reward system.

Then what I want you to do is put on three songs – just three. And rather than timing your exercises with a stopwatch, or by the amount of reps, you're going to use the verse and chorus of each song as your guide to switch up your exercises. Here's what I mean . . .

Song 1:
First verse – rest
Chorus – hold plank
Second verse – rest
Chorus – plank
Middle eight – rest
Last chorus – plank!

Song 2:
First verse – wall squat
Chorus – punch the air above you
Second verse – wall squat
Chorus – punch the air in front of you
Middle eight – wall squat
Last chorus – punch the air above . . .

Song 3:
First verse – stand on one leg
Chorus – walking lunges
Second verse – stand on other leg
Chorus – walking lunges
Middle eight – stand on first leg again
Last chorus – walking lunges . . .

You should do this every single day, and, over time, begin to improve how long you can hold movements for. It's not about aiming for a world-record plank but holding it for five more seconds than you did last week. Little by little. Add on a track or two as you build strength. Add more exercises. Sing along if you like! And take notes so you can see the speed of your progress.

By exercising to uplifting music, you're shaping it around dopamine release, which will make you feel better and motivate you to push through the burn. This is a real gateway workout that will make you feel more positive and start that muscle synthesis process.

To do from home: get rucking

Rucking has become a super-fashionable exercise in recent years, especially in California, because as we all know, these super-healthy US types *love* to go on a three-hour hike with their mates. (Though if I'm being honest, I can't imagine anything worse than being stuck with someone for three hours up a mountain, but each to their own.)

Simply put, rucking is walking while carrying a weighted rucksack/backpack. This increased weight turns what might be a nice little cardio burst into muscle-building exercise – focusing on your legs, core and that hard-to-reach back and shoulder area.[23] It has its roots in military training, which is probably why it's been taken up by all these biohacking blokes as the latest thing; but really, anyone can get started with rucking. You don't even need to buy one of the specially weighted rucking backpacks; just fill your usual backpack with loads of bottles of water! That way, you'll have plenty to drink on your ruck in any case.

Rucking is ridiculously easy to get started with and it is a great way to get your outdoor mood-boosting sunlight, too.

(Remember that you benefit from vitamin D exposure even when it's cloudy.) I wasn't brought up in a walking family, so I have to make a bit more of an effort now to build it into my life, but really it is a fabulous skill set to have, and gets kids out in nature, too. So load up your backpack with water, or even bags of rice, small handweights or books. Go on an outdoors walk from forty minutes to an hour, and the contraction and expansion of muscles as you walk up and down inclines will fat burn, support bone density and build muscle, even though you don't realise it. And remember, just wee in a bush if you need – a 'wild wee' I've heard it called!

To do from home: electrical muscle stimulation (EMS)

Yes, I hear you say, wait, *what?* EMS, which is sometimes called electrical myostimulation, is indeed the use of electrical currents to improve muscle function. It has been proven to be absolutely brilliant results-wise, helping with both building muscle and reducing muscle atrophy (sarcopenia).[24] After all, we humans are electrical beings, constantly sending electrical messages around our body through our nervous system.[25] It's why defibrillators work in bringing us back to life!

How does it work?
EMS works by mimicking the impulse that comes from our central nervous system during exercise, causing our muscles to contract. It does this by sending safe electrical currents throughout our body via electrodes. There are a few different ways you can do it – via an EMS suit, toning belts, or even a TENS machine (that those of us who have given birth may remember very well from throwing across a delivery suite . . .)

Who is this good for?

EMS can increase muscle strength and is recommended as a kick start protocol, rather than a permanent solution. So, if you've never exercised or have a mental block, you could try this as a first step rather than waste your time trying to work out with a tin of tomatoes. It's also a great way in for older people, those who are bedbound or recovering from illness and surgery as it's fast, safe, comfortable and has no injury risk.

It's also an excellent option if you want to maximise your results. I recently tried out an EMS suit when I was at a longevity clinic and found the experience fabulous! I wore it while I did a workout and it conducted electricity throughout my whole body. This increased my fat-burning and muscle-building, so I didn't mind looking like a bit of a dick while I wore it.

How do I get started?

You can buy EMS suits for use at home. The prices can really vary. A good option is either to hunt a cheap one down on eBay or rent them via a gym or supplier – which is a good idea as they are not meant for permanent use. It's all about waking up your muscle memory even if you haven't exercised for decades. Alternatively, you can book on to an EMS class that is run by an instructor.

Some helpful benchmark goals

It's really difficult to set universal goals; after all, we're different ages, different sizes and at different levels of fitness. However, I did come across this really helpful set of targets for physical fitness for forty-year-olds from Dr Peter Attia. According to him, this is what we should be aiming for:

Dead hangs:	1½ minutes (women)	2 minutes (men)
Air squat at 90 degrees:	2 minutes (both sexes)	
Farmer's carry (holding weights on either side):	75 per cent body weight (women)	100 per cent body weight (men)

You'll be surprised how quickly your body hits these targets – we're talking weeks not months!

Some great muscle-building supplements

Vitamin D is vital for reducing musculoskeletal pain. If you are deficient, then lower levels of calcium are absorbed, and you are more likely to have bone pain and sarcopenia. So if you feel muscular pain, feel weak and fatigued, you could do a lot worse than add in a vitamin D supplement. A good daily dose is 15mcg and it should be taken with MK-7 (a more active form of vitamin K) and magnesium.

Tart cherry extract has been scientifically proven to reduce delayed-onset muscle soreness (DOMS), which is the aching you normally feel a couple of days after exercising strenuously.[26] It has anti-inflammatory properties as well as loads of vitamins and minerals, so is a great choice for improved muscle-recovery time – either in extract or juice format.[27] A good daily dose is 500mg.

Magnesium sulphate is another great one for post-muscle workout recovery because it is vital for protein synthesis (more to come on that in the next chapter!), which reduces muscle soreness post training the next day. A lovely night-time tip is to buy a spray version which you can spray on your feet before bed.[28] (Please note this one isn't for oral consumption!)

Creatine is a compound of amino acids naturally found in the body and is now commonly taken as a supplement to build muscle mass. It works because it improves the hydration of your muscle cells, which increases power output by around 12–20 per cent and therefore powers muscle growth. Numerous studies have confirmed how effective it is, so it's become hugely popular as a workout supplement.[29] You can get creatine from red meat and chicken, but you'd have to eat a large amount and this is no good if you're vegetarian obviously, so supplements are recommended. It has an outstanding safety profile and around 3–5g daily is a recommended dose, depending on your weight.

Salt is a very misunderstood mineral, and I can really recommend *The Salt Fix* by Dr James DiNicolantonio if you'd like to take a deep dive into it. It's actually recommended to take on *more* salt, before and after exercise, to replenish electrolytes lost in sweating and aid muscle-building (unless of course you're on medication which has a cautionary warning on salt intake).[30] Don't forget, we are made of salt! All isotonic sports energy drinks are salty, because they increase fluid and energy absorption, but they're packed with sugar and additives, so I'd avoid them. You can take a small dose of salt and then quickly rinse your mouth out for a super-cheap and easy salt boost. When buying electrolytes, look for products that use stevia or allulose as a sweetener, rather than standard sugar and sucralose.

Why I'm still challenging myself

I'm very conscious that I'm coming up to fifty, and I need to focus on muscle mass for my own longevity. Recently I got my skeletal muscle mass score assessed, which was 20.69kg. This is high, especially for someone my age, which is great because it means I'm on the right track. I love my running and I'm not going to give that up, because it's so great for meditative purposes and clearing my head. But moving into the next few decades of my life, I want to know that I'm a strong, robust, resilient woman; and that confidence will lie in building protective muscle, so I will continue to up my muscle work in the gym.

Until recently, I hadn't realised that building muscle wasn't just about strength, but was integral to healthy lifespan, and to protect us from injury, disease and mental illness. I do now, so there's no excuse. So these days, I'm working out in the gym like a lad – for the gains! That means taking notes, writing down what my one-rep max is. I'm pushing myself by working on my areas of weakness, which is my abs and my arms. I've always wanted to be able to do proper pull-ups, which I'd never been able to do because I've got a really crappy grip.

DOES GRIP STRENGTH REALLY MATTER?

Grip strength is regularly used as a biomarker for ageing as it supposedly measures your overall strength, upper-limb function, bone density, etc., etc.[31] However, I've always been a bit suspicious about its reliability as a measure of longevity; because if you have a bigger hand and longer fingers, then surely you will be able to grip harder and longer than somebody with small, short tendons? I was told years ago by my PT Charlie that I had the grip strength of a toddler – but then again, that was when I was on calorie control, so no wonder I was weak and feeble!

In any case, my stupid little witchy child fingers aren't long enough to wrap around a bar for long enough to do proper chin-ups or deadlifts. If I hang off *anything*, I find my grip is crap and sweaty and I just slide off. To hack this, I've started using a piece of very cheap kit called weight-lifting hooks. You can buy them for not much more than a tenner off Amazon: they have a flexible strap that wraps around your wrists, then a rigid, curved hook that you curve your fingers over. If you've got a rubbish grip, it means that part doesn't let you down because the hook looks after that, and you can focus on the lifting and muscle-building!

MY TOP FIVE MUSCLE-BOOSTING TAKEAWAYS

Whatever sounds interesting to you, I encourage you just to try it. Even if it's been years and years since you trained, do not worry. We have a great thing called muscle memory. Scientific research now shows that this is a genuine thing – our cells hold on to the epigenetic 'recipe' for how to do something.[32] Even if it's been decades since you climbed a tree or a fence, your muscle memory is phenomenal and will kick in. So you *will* build muscle because your body has always known how to do it. It will release the right enzymes and proteins, and you *will* get stronger.

1. **Join a gym:** Rethink your perception of the gym and look for one which will stop you making excuses to get there – it's your key to real muscle gains.
2. **Create a power playlist:** and make working out dopamine-fuelled.
3. **Commit to ten minutes a day:** for your home-based muscle-building exercises.
4. **Log your one-rep max:** and track your progress each week.
5. **It's never too late:** you can start wherever, whenever. So remember, progress not perfection!

FUTUREPROOF PRINCIPLE #3: EAT FOR VITALITY

How I used to eat for 'energy' . . .

When I look back at what I used to eat to sustain me, I'm like, *frigging hell, no wonder I was knackered!* I was completely driven by that low-fat, low-calorie panic, so my diet was full of virtue-signalling salads, with their low-fat salad dressing, super-lean meat, whole grains and brown bread. There was very little fat, because we all thought 'fat makes you fat' (which of course it doesn't, it's just spelled the same!). So, when the Japanese-style food craze kicked off during the 1990s and 2000s, me and my mates were absolutely thrilled: here were teeny-tiny salads and piddly bits of fish glazed in a sugary coating, which we all thought it was *so healthy* because the fat content was on the floor! No matter that the reality of eating this stuff meant I'd end up gorging on pizzas and butties in private later, because I was absolutely starving ... craving ... craving ... *What is wrong with me*, I'd think? I'm never satisfied!

I certainly *never* considered the role of protein. To be honest, I used to mentally park protein in the just-for-blokes category, because of steak being a stereotypical 'man thing', men drinking protein shakes at the gym, my grandad being a fan of meat and two veg, all of that. It wasn't of interest to me in any way, shape or form, so I completely neglected that side of my eating. For me, in my addicted, misinformed state, it was always about the bread. I was, and remain, a complete (recovering) carb addict! So, there you go, that was me then, relying on a bottle of wine and some toast to keep me going ... (huge eye rolls, here) and thinking isn't red meat for uneducated fools who want cancer, obviously???

. . . Why it was so wrong . . .

There was so much I thought I knew that was utterly wrong. I thought carbs were the perfect, preferred 'energy source' for the body, because that's the narrative I grew up with. Carbs equal energy equal get-up-and-go, right? It turns out that information I was given was wrong – the body only uses carbs for energy because high blood sugar is super-toxic, so they have to try and get rid of it first. And I didn't know that unless you immediately went on a huge long-distance run to burn all of them off, those carbs just converted to fat and sat on your bum, belly and back of your arms. (Sidebar – have you seen just how long you'd need to stay on a treadmill to burn off the energy from one finger of KitKat? And who eats just one finger, which is the so-called 'portion size'? Madness! *Anyway*.)

I didn't know that upping my protein intake would not only satisfy me and curb my cravings via steadying my blood sugar, but also help me build muscle, stability and better mental health. I had no idea it had any particular use in my body. There was *so much* I didn't know.

. . . And how I eat now

Cut to nowadays. If I need a snack, my first port of call is some scrambled eggs, made with cheese and butter. If I've got some avocado, or some smoked salmon (ideally wild, not farmed) with a squeeze of lemon, I'll have them, too. By the time I've eaten and given it a while to digest, and for those hormonal satiety signals to travel from my gut to my brain, I'll have a think. Do I want something else? If so, do you know what? I'll have a protein shake. Usually, I won't need anything more, because the protein in those eggs has sorted me out, as have the good saturated fats in the avocado, too.

That's now my 'break in case of emergency' hunger protocol. It used to be biscuits, and now it's that. Look, I still hate washing up the scrambled-egg pan afterwards, but it's way better than how I used to be: battling the immediate craving for sweet things that would kick off as soon as I walked through the front door, and the carb coma that followed, which means no sugar or breads. I always make sure I have good-quality protein in the house like eggs, meat and cheese for this reason – I am a hungry person, I love my food and my eyes are often bigger than my tummy!

I've learned so much fascinating information about just how vital what we eat is, and how we've got the nutritional balance the wrong way around. Not for dieting, or for losing weight, but for longevity. In this chapter, you'll learn about how we can futureproof ourselves with the food we eat, what to add in and what to reduce, why red meat isn't the enemy and why 'superfoods' aren't all they're cracked up to be. We'll also take a deep dive into skin health and how to age well without filler and Botox.

WHAT IS PROTEIN, AND WHAT DOES IT DO?

Protein is so important. It's a macronutrient essential for the growth, repair and maintenance of various tissues in the human body. It plays so many essential roles, powering biological functions like our hormones, immune system, structural support and muscle development. I'll dive more into how protein and muscle work together in a bit, but just know that muscle is simply one piece of the amazing protein puzzle . . . Our bones, ligaments, tendons, liver, brain, skin and fingernails are all made from proteins, too! It literally builds us. So, we all need protein for the structure, metabolic function and regulation of our tissues and organs.

Dr Gabrielle Lyon, who wrote the *Forever Strong* book I mentioned earlier, is a huge fan, explaining that 'protein is involved in virtually every one of our cellular functions'. Give that a moment to sink in: protein is critically important because we need it to actually function! For this reason, our bodies constantly need new supplies of it from the food we eat. However, protein's *bioavailability* – which basically means how effectively it can be absorbed and used by the body – can vary massively. It completely depends on what you eat, how you eat it and its amino-acid profile.

HANG ON – WHAT ARE AMINO ACIDS?

If you follow me on Instagram, or have read any of my previous books, you'll have heard me talk about amino acids a lot. In a nutshell, amino acids are small molecules that are used to build proteins. Therefore, they're commonly referred to as the 'building blocks of life'.[1]

Amino acids are either *essential, non-essential* or *conditional.* Non-essential amino acids are the ones that our bodies can make themselves, even if we don't get them from food. Conditional ones are those we only need when we're ill. Essential amino acids – the ones we really should focus on – are the ones we *need* to get from our food, because our bodies cannot make them otherwise. Simple, right?

OK, now the not-so-simple. The nine essential amino acids are: histidine, isoleucine, leucine, lysine, methionine, phenylalanine, threonine, tryptophan and valine. Don't worry, you do not need to remember these names! However, it's probably worth noting the three 'branched-chain' amino acids, which are *leucine, valine* and *isoleucine.* These form a supergroup of essential amino acids, and leucine in particular plays a key role in building muscle, preventing muscle wastage and regulating our blood-sugar levels. (Which we will look at *again* in a bit – I know, but honestly, it is utterly vital in preserving longevity.)

Forgetting all these medical terms for a moment, though, what's essential knowledge is that *our bodies need a full amino-*

acid profile from our food – otherwise many of our bodily functions simply won't work properly. For example, that crazy hunger we get an hour after eating loads of toast or a tube of Pringles? That's because that crappy 'food' didn't contain anywhere near a full complement of amino acids, so our poor bodies send out desperate hormonal signals for *more, more, more* – leading to overeating, weight gain and all the horrible cascade of effects we've explored before (and for more on appetite and amino acids, my last book, *Hack Your Hormones*, covers this). Not to mention, these addicting foods are full of ingredients that seem to have been designed by mathematicians, not dietitians, in order to be the most addictive as possible for maximum and repeat sales. We need to empower ourselves to supercharge our diets with foods that are protein-rich, bioavailable, and that will give our bodies the full amino-acid profile they need in order to work their magic.

THE AMAZING ROLES OF COLLAGEN

This is a great place for us to talk about collagen, which is another wonder molecule. It's a small protein made up of amino acids, which obviously we are all experts in now! (Ahem.) We have collagen everywhere, and it is the most abundant protein in our body as it structurally supports our connective tissues.[2] It's particularly present in the deep layers of our skin – making up 70 per cent of its overall protein.

Collagen is fabulous because it works as a type of scaffolding, holding things in place all over our body. It also has a role in looking after our (takes deep breath) bones, skin, teeth, muscles, cartilage, tendons, ligaments, arteries and even intestinal health – bolstering the tight junctions and maintaining the integrity of our gut lining, which, as we saw earlier on, is vitally important. It keeps our bones and joints sturdy, and our hair, nails and skin in top condition, especially when we're young and full of natural collagen. (I'll go a bit more into our skin health and collagen later on.)

Glorious glycine

There are loads of different amino acids that make up collagen, but the main one we want to focus on is *glycine*. Glycine makes up a third of our total collagen and is an absolutely incredible amino acid. It has all sorts of super-jobs to do: synthesising oestrogen, fighting off oxidative stress and reducing inflammation, promoting cell growth, creating bile salts which help digest and break down fats, getting rid of ammonia, reducing inflammation – the list just goes on! It is especially brilliant for our skin, too – lots more on this later.

So, hurrah for collagen and its myriad health benefits. But although collagen renewal constantly takes place, like most things, its rate depletes over time: we have less collagen as we get older. However, do not worry. We can help restore our declining collagen levels by adding it back into our bodies, via collagen-rich and collagen-promoting foods, and supplementing with collagen powder.

Boosting the benefits

Adding in collagen peptides to our diet has been found to be incredibly beneficial. Although it's an 'incomplete' protein source – it's missing tryptophan and therefore doesn't have the full amino-acid profile – studies have found it offers real health improvements.[3] It can improve our skin's elasticity, repair cartilage, strengthen tendons and ligaments, improve lean muscle mass and reduce pain. What's more, it increases bone-mineral density in post-menopausal women and thereby helps guard against osteoporosis.[4]

Even better, if you're following a keto-style plan, you can add collagen supplements into your drinks and remain in a fat-fasted state, as it won't spike your blood sugar. I am a huge fan of collagen powder and MCT oil and am forever adding it into my coffees, cold drinks, soups and stews. Sneaking that nutrition in and supporting glycine synthesis wherever I can!

FUTUREPROOFING OURSELVES WITH PROTEIN

Our bodies only work at their best if we fuel them with the right nutrients. As Dr Mark Hyman puts it, food is the 'master controller' of longevity, switching on the right functions and helping us feel good and thriving. Or the opposite. I know first-hand just how awful you can feel and look if you're eating all the wrong things, something which Dr Gabrielle has also experienced. In her book, she writes about being obsessed with weight loss in her past and relying on carbs for energy, which left her not only starving hungry, but 'exhausted and malnourished'. Yep, me too. She transformed her outlook and her health by introducing high-quality protein into her diet, and I've done the same.

What's more, it's vitally important that we increase our protein intake as we age – often the received wisdom is that we need less, but this is an utter myth. As we'll see, **protein is a vital component of all our longevity protocols** as it fights so many of the damaging hallmarks of ageing and disease. We need to consume protein faster than our bodies are breaking it down to maintain a healthy future.

PRO-PROTEIN REASON #1: IT FIGHTS INSULIN RESISTANCE

As we age, we're more likely to be insulin resistant, which is a shitshow for our healthspan in so many ways. We've already seen how insulin resistance can spark disease through inflammation, and the number one culprit for this is our carb-heavy diet: eating too much bread, pasta, crisps, fizzy drinks and most UPFs. I know I've already covered this before, but in case you need a quick recap as to *why* this happens, here goes:

- Carbs break down into sugar in our bloodstream.
- This elevates our blood-glucose levels.
- Our bodies release insulin to bring this level down.
- Insulin takes glucose from our blood to our cells for energy.
- Blood-sugar levels reduce.

However, the more and more we overconsume carbs, and the more and more insulin we produce, the more we become resistant to its effects. High blood sugar is really dangerous and toxic to our cells (just see the horrendous diseases caused by diabetes), so the body will rush in immediately to burn it first. If we have too much, the body ends up storing the excess sugar as fat in our cells, because it has to store it somewhere, leading to slower metabolism, cravings, weight gain and inflammation – as well as a cascade of diseases.

Insulin resistance is a huge issue we can't ignore if we want a healthy lifespan, so switching up what we eat is a great way to tackle it. By upping our intake of protein and good fats, we'll give ourselves all the nutrition we need, without so much of the insulin spike. I'll set out some simple meal ideas with protein-boosting foods later in this chapter.

Years ago, when I was stacking my diet with carbs, I believed that I had to keep my blood-sugar levels up because it gave me energy. (Absolute balls.) I had no idea that in fact it was depleting me; and instead my poor insulin was skyrocketing in the background while it tried to dampen down my elevated glucose levels.

So, you may think that this advice doesn't apply to you – especially if you've had your glucose levels checked and had them come back 'normal'. That doesn't mean you're fine, because glucose levels do not tell you about your insulin levels, which could be working overtime in the background trying to keep blood glucose down. Blood glucose and insulin are two different measurements. Your insulin could be going completely haywire and you'd never know, because measuring your glucose is cheaper, faster and easier for GPs. A fasting insulin test is a great way to see if somebody is prediabetic, which would end up saving the NHS money in the long run!

What's more, if you're of an average weight, you might find the doctors are resistant to check you *anyway* because you're not ticking the risk boxes for obesity. Behind the scenes, you could be knackered, headed for depression, insulin resistance and diabetes, not to mention everything else – but you'll be told you're 'healthy' because your BMI is within a certain threshold! Or you don't have prediabetes, even though thirty years ago you would have been told you do (the 'healthy' range for fasting glucose levels has risen considerably from 65–85mg/dl to 70–100mg/dl). It's certainly not the full picture. However, the NHS is so stretched, we need to take care of this ourselves. And we can reduce the risk by moving towards a more protein-rich, nutritionally dense eating plan.

PRO-PROTEIN REASON #2: IT SUPPORTS MUSCLE GROWTH

Protein and muscles are completely symbiotic. They work brilliantly together and complement each other in a beautiful partnership. We can't have one without the other – e.g. we won't build muscle without protein. This is because, unlike carbs, both protein and fat have loads of *other* jobs to do in our bodies, one of which is to help build muscle. As Dr Mark puts it, to build muscle, we need to eat muscle.

This is because we need that full complement of amino acids in our protein to kick-start our protein-muscle synthesis, where the body turns the nutrients from protein into muscle cells. As we know, building more muscle as we age is vitally important in staving off sarcopenia, the process of depleted muscle mass which can be a disaster zone for older people. But we can't resistance-train effectively if we're just eating crisps and biscuits. We need to consume high-quality protein with the right amino-acid profile in order to activate protein synthesis and help us build stability, strength and security.

Eating more protein is fantastic if we're trying to lose weight as well. Firstly, because having more muscle mass means we become a metabolic furnace! We burn off that excess energy much more effectively than carbs. Secondly – and which leads me on to my next point . . .

PRO-PROTEIN REASON #3: IT KEEPS US FULLER FOR LONGER

Eating a higher-protein diet has been proven to increase the sensation of satiety (fullness) and reduce food cravings.[5] Our brains and bodies are constantly seeking those essential amino acids from our food so that they can restore and regenerate. If we eat a fantastic diet full of bioavailable proteins containing that full amino-acid profile, then bingo! As soon as our brain registers this and they're in our system, it switches off those hunger hormones and stops us feeling that desperate craving for more food. I add a teaspoon of collagen to each of my drinks to give myself those amino acids, which gives my brain the immediate signal that all is fine, I do not need a brownie. Remember the gut–brain axis – and the gut starts in the mouth!

Not only that, but as protein and fats don't mess with our glucose levels as much as carbs, we don't experience those horrendous sugar crashes that also trigger the sensation of hunger. In this way, eating more protein dampens down that subliminal seeking that can plague us as we're constantly surrounded by temptation – the advertising and high-street fast-food outlets that make us buy and eat shit! It's really a win–win all round.

THE LONGEVITY DISASTER ZONE OF OUR MODERN DIET

So much damage has been done to our overall health outcomes with our super-processed Western diet. We simply can't carry on the way we have been if we want to live an optimal life – it's time to take off the rose-tinted glasses about just what 'convenience' food and an obsession with low calories is doing to us. When I think about it, it's *nuts* – we have simply forgotten how to eat properly, the way our grandparents did, using simple whole foods cooked from scratch!

Not only that, but I believe we all need to question the advice that's fed to us on what constitutes 'healthy eating'. So much of what's out there, and passed along to us via our GPs, schools and government campaigns, is just plain *wrong*.

FLIPPING THE THINKING – WHY 'HEALTHY EATING' ISN'T HEALTHY

Even before I started biohacking, and reading up about the science behind our biology, hormones and food, I could have told you that the 'healthy eating' advice I was given was bullshit. Because it simply *didn't work*.

Take a look at the UK government's Eatwell Guide, or the food pyramid if you're in the US. These official guidelines tell us that we should fill up on wholegrains, cut down on fat and watch our calorie intakes like a hawk. The Eatwell Guide recommends that almost 40 per cent of our diet should come from starchy carbs like potatoes, pasta and bread. That we should minimise protein to only around 12 per cent of our diet and avoid red meat. That we shouldn't eat butter, but instead use veg-oil-packed margarines. That we should be monitoring our calorie intake to 2,000 a day for women, 2,500 for men.[6] This is supposed to represent a 'balanced' diet!

Years ago, I followed all this advice to the letter. I ended up overweight, inflamed and depressed. I mean, it's no wonder! All those carbs were instantly converting to glucose, and spiking my insulin constantly. I wasn't building strong muscle as I didn't have the right protein intake (and was frankly too bloody tired to work out). I was frustrated – if I was doing all the 'healthy' things, then how come I felt so unhealthy, depleted and also really flipping hungry all the time? At this point I didn't even drink alcohol at all but felt hung-over every day, with brain fog, lack of enthusiasm and zero patience and tolerance.

OK, what happened with me is my own personal story and it's not scientific research – although there are plenty of studies out there now to back up and explain why I felt like I did. But I hear similar stories every single day, from the thousands of my followers who get in touch via Instagram. They are sick and tired (*literally*) of following the so-called healthy-eating advice out there and feeling worse than ever. However, the thousands of stories across the globe are still not enough evidence to stop the rhetoric of the high-carb/low-fat religion of all the major advisory boards, many of which are influenced by the American Heart Association guidelines, which I believe is the most powerful organisation on the planet when it comes to dietary influence. They insist on low saturated fat and high grain regardless of the downstream effects on other systems in the body.

What's going on with this? Why are we being advised to load our diet full of foods that drive insulin resistance and promote obesity? I think it's worth noting that the panel that formulated this guide were primarily members of the food and drink industry, *not* independent health experts.[7] Food companies make the most money on foods that are the cheapest to produce (that'll be grains, then). And it's not just me – experts have described this guide as being designed for 'wealth, not health' as it has *no* positive impact on reducing obesity or type 2 diabetes.[8] In fact, the panel who were brought together by Public Health England to review the Eatwell Guide in the UK in 2014 was not made up of experts at all. Instead, it was packed full of representatives from the worst fake-food associations in the country, such as the Association of Convenience Stores and the British Nutrition Foundation (whose members include Coca-Cola, Danone, PepsiCo and McDonald's). (Zoe Harcombe has written extensively about this and I encourage you to read her articles on the conflict of interest inherent in the creation of the Eatwell Guide.[9])

What these guides suggest is the literal opposite of what I've found to be true. I only transformed my health, both mentally and physically, when I flipped these guidelines upside down. Once I started eating *more* high-quality protein and fats that nourished my brain and body and *less* of the starchy carbs. Once I learned that it's not just wholemeal bread that gives you fibre – you can get the same amount of fibre from an avocado![10] And once I stopped counting calories . . .

It's no wonder people are confused about what to eat when most dieticians promote things like overnight oats as a great, 'sustaining' breakfast – whereas the truth is that they convert instantly to sugar, stop you burning fat and leave you starving. When they're advised to carb-load for 'energy' when it leaves us sluggish, inflamed and ill. I passionately believe that this wholegrain obsession needs to go. We have to get our heads around the truth: we need to eat fewer carbs, but more protein and more good fats. We'll be satisfied, healthier and more resilient. More futureproof.

FLIPPING THE THINKING – THE TOXIC SO-CALLED SUPERFOODS

Do you remember what happened to Liam Hemsworth a few years ago? The completely ripped, super-buff movie star? He got kidney stones because of too many oxalates in his vegan diet.[11] Yep, his daily green smoothie, with spinach, almonds, plant milk and vegan protein powder was chock full of toxicity that made him properly ill, and ultimately led him to 'completely reconsider' the diet he thought was super-healthy. Sounds crazy, but it's true – these so-called superfoods can cause us harm!

What are oxalates, then?
Oxalate is an organic acid molecule, which we usually get rid of as a by-product of metabolism. We can produce oxalates on our own or from the foods we eat – and certain plants are very high in oxalates because they use them to store their own energy. It's a fact that some vegetables, like spinach or Swiss chard, are incredibly high in oxalates, which have been proven to cause kidney stones and make

it more difficult for your body to absorb minerals, too.[12]

It won't surprise you to know that I have a huge question mark over the plant-based obsession of the last few years. Yes, of course there are some benefits to be had from eating more vegetables, but overpacking our diets with plants and processed fake meats at the expense of real protein and fats to be found in proper food? *Nope.* I mean, did your great-grandma drink green smoothies? No, she did not! And the idea that spinach is full of iron is a complete fiction. (Apparently the reason the cartoon character Popeye was originally given spinach as a 'source' of his amazing strength was down to a missed decimal point – a scientist reported it as containing 35mg of iron per serving rather than 3.5mg – this led to the long-standing misconception that it is full of iron when it's not![13])

Easy swaps and the one supplement to reduce oxalates

If you suffer from UTIs, or are susceptible to kidney stones or kidney disease, try reducing your oxalate-dense foods or swapping them out for an alternative. Look, if you're completely in love with the taste of spinach (I mean, someone out there *must* like it) you don't need to ditch it entirely, but don't eat too much – don't do your kidneys a disservice. Here are a few easy exchanges to reduce your oxalate load.[14]

Swap	*For*
Spinach (raw or cooked)	Rocket (much nicer anyway!)
Rhubarb	Bananas
Swiss chard	Pak choi

Baked potatoes	Mashed celeriac
Sweet potatoes	Butternut squash
Pre-made tomato sauce	Fresh tomatoes

There are hundreds more examples of high-oxalate foods that can easily be found online. Overall, though, soy products are another high-oxalate food, whereas meat and cheese are fine, so vegans and vegetarians need to be extra-careful here. But spinach and chard really are the worst offenders – which is good news for you and your kids, because you don't need to feel guilty any more about trying to get them to eat them!

Another useful hack to reduce your risk of oxalates is to get yourself a **magnesium oxide supplement** – studies have suggested that it may decrease intestinal absorption of oxalate, and also helps it leave the body quicker through our urine.[15] However, you have to take it *without food* to maximise its benefits. Another way is through a sparkling magnesium drink like OHMG. This mineral is found in natural water and brings us all sorts of benefits like improved sleep and immunity, better brain health and less stress.[16] However, in the absence of a bubbling spring to get our water from, we need to add it back in ourselves!

Think protein-first, not carb-first

I hope by now I've managed to arm you with enough knowledge and encouragement to make protein a priority. Along with natural saturated fats, which we explored in the inflammation chapter, they provide a myriad of great benefits for our bodies and minds. They help build muscles, bones, enzymes, neurotransmitters, hormones and our cell membranes – as well as provide us with energy. Carbs can't do all those things. And, as Dr Mark Hyman points out: 'below the neck your body doesn't know the difference between a fizzy drink and a bagel' – as far as our biochemical processes are concerned, it's *all* sugar!

So, the best thing we can do with our diet to maintain longevity is reduce refined carbs and add in plenty of essential proteins and fats. Of course, I'm not asking you to eliminate carbs entirely – we're working with reality, here! I'm just asking you to think protein-first, not carb-first. It's swapping the focus from one to the other. I promise, you will feel satisfied and will slowly start to let go of that addictive craving.

This isn't about restriction, this is about adding in, about abundance, about foods that taste great and do us good. About more Greek yogurt, more eggs, more beef! And not about eating faddy foods that deplete us. Because life *is* too short for that kale smoothie which just makes you paranoid about farting and nobody needs yet another thing to worry about.

HOW MUCH PROTEIN SHOULD I HAVE?

There are so many different guidelines out there on how to calculate your 'optimal' amount of protein. Some advice recommends aiming for around 25g–40g protein per meal. But others put it differently. One guideline is to have a minimum daily amount of 0.8g per kilogram of body weight,[17] but if you're older (than what?) you need between 1.5g and 2g per kg per day. Then there are others who say you need up to 1.7g if you're training, and yet *another* that reckons it's 1–1.25g of protein per pound of lean body weight. I mean, WTF is your 'lean' body weight? Mine must be less than my actual body weight of about 62kg, but how am I supposed to know what that is? And then there's the stress of converting kilos to pounds . . . argh!

Quite frankly, I find all these numbers a bit too sciency and unhelpful. They just overwhelm and confuse me, so it doesn't work for me to sit there fiddling around with a calculator. From my perspective, and I reckon for many of us, the better option is to listen to our bodies. To eat until we're full, and then stop. Let's get intuitive about this. We don't need stats from a scientist or some gym dude – I mean, how they even work this stuff out, God only knows! And it's ridiculous to claim that every single cohort will be the same just based on their body weight. Our appetites and needs chop and change all the time, depending on all sorts of factors: our mental energy, how cold it is outside, not to mention the impact from the menstrual cycle for women of certain age ranges . . . There are all *sorts* of shifts.

So I say: eat to satisfaction. Then, give it fifteen minutes before you eat anything else to know whether you're properly full or not. Let's learn to listen our bodies. It only takes a couple of weeks to start feeling the difference.

PROTEIN-PACKED SUPERHEROES

There are so many different protein sources we can add into our diet. Although some protein powders are great – but not all, which I'll get to – it's always best to get your main protein source from whole foods rather than supplements. The following foods are known for being brilliant sources of dietary protein, and I've given you an average serving size for each (aside from eggs . . .)

Beef steak (150g serving)	35g
Chicken thigh with the skin on (130g)	31g[18]
Grilled salmon fillet (120g)	27g
Cod (120g)	20g
Greek yogurt (200g)	20g[19]
Tempeh (fermented soy, 125g)	20g
Chickpeas (100g)	19g
Cottage cheese (125g)	12g
Lentils (125g)	9g
Hemp seeds (30g)	9g[20]
Cheddar cheese (30g)	7.6g
Pumpkin seeds (30g)	7.3g
Peanut butter (but watch out for its veg-oil content) (2 tbsp)	7g
One large egg	6g
Nuts (e.g. Brazil, walnuts, 30g)	5g
Quinoa (125g, cooked)	4g
White rice, cooked and cooled increases resistant starch) (100g)	2.7g
New potatoes (100g)	2g

MEALS AND SNACKS TO AMP UP YOUR PROTEIN

Of course, if we're going to go protein-first rather than carb-first, we need some ideas on how to do that. Not all of us are brilliant cooks, but it's very easy to make some simple recipes that prioritise protein and good fats. It's clear from the table above that meat and fish are super-easy ways to get a fabulous dose of protein, but I know that can get expensive (coming from someone who did a month on the carnivore plan recently!). A good approach would be to combine plant with animal proteins, so you not only get a variety of different foods in your diet but also keep it affordable. I found that I saved money overall in my first year of doing this as over time I ate less due to regulating my appetite.

Here are just a few to get you started, along with rough information about the general protein count in each. (This will of course vary depending on the size of your portion, and how you cook it.)

Meal ideas

Steak with quinoa and rocket – 40g
Grilled salmon fillet with lentils and veg – 36g
Roasted cod with chickpeas and tomatoes – 39g
Three-egg omelette with cheese – 24g
Tempeh with stir-fried rice and veg – 22g

Snacks

Greek yogurt with hemp seeds and walnuts – 34g
Peanut butter on sourdough toast – 10g
Protein shake (made with water) – 16g
Cottage cheese and sprinkling of pumpkin seeds – 15g

WHAT'S THE DIFFERENCE BETWEEN ANIMAL AND PLANT PROTEINS?

The simple fact is that it's harder to boost your protein intake if you're vegetarian or vegan. Just look at the charts above and you can see how much more protein you get from meat, poultry, fish and dairy. What's more, animal and plant proteins are *not the same*. Animal proteins are highly bioavailable, because they contain all the essential amino acids that our bodies need. Meat proteins contain high levels of leucine and creatine, too, which are vital for muscle-building and brain health.

This isn't the case with plant proteins. With the exception of quinoa and hemp seeds, they don't have a complete amino-acid profile. Also, unlike animal products, they don't have proper source traceability – you can't be sure how they are harvested or what their provenance is. Saying something is 'plant-based' doesn't mean it's been ethically manufactured or without the use of pesticides! Look at the hazmat suits they wear in some parts of the world when they are spraying pesticides on fruit and veg. It really drives home that this is profit above quality in our food-supply systems.

What's more, the protein from plant sources is often not well absorbed by the body, so the protein they do contain can't be used. They're just not nutrient-dense enough, and Dr Mark Hyman describes them as 'inadequate', so it's not just me! I know I have a reputation as being anti-vegan, but it's actually the mis-selling of veganism as the 'healthier' approach that really riles me. It's just not true – the stats bear me out and you will struggle to hit a satisfactory protein level on a vegan diet.

I understand that, of course, lots of people are vegetarian for religious reasons, and in those cases, I would recommend really leaning into the dairy: eat plenty of cheese and Greek yogurt, eggs and sprinkle hemp seeds over whatever you can. (And by the way, if you are sensitive to dairy, you might want to have a look at raw dairy as opposed to pasteurised, which boils out all the digestive enzymes which can be better tolerated. Goat's milk is another good option – so maybe give it a go.)

I completely get that loads of you are reluctant to eat meat, too, because of the horrendous industrialised farming methods that go on in this country, so decide not to for ethical or environmental reasons. But we can take the guilt and the shame out of this by getting to know the practices of our local farmers and supporting them by buying their meat instead. And by God, do farmers need us lot back on their doorstep!

This is not only better for the environment (thanks to regenerative farming), but better for us, because grass-fed meat is more nutrient-dense. Look, most of us reading this live in bloody Britain and Ireland where it pisses down with rain all the time, so at least we've got the best grass in the world! This means all the ruminant animals (cows, sheep and goats) who graze on it are fantastically nutrient-dense. Even if you don't live near a farm, you can get a delivery of frozen meat from a farm supplier pretty much everywhere in the country now. And this gives us something to do with that air fryer (hopefully a glass or stainless steel one as opposed to non-stick or Teflon) or slow cooker that's sitting on our kitchen worktops, doesn't it? We can chuck that good meat into it! So, eat local, support small producers and try and cut out the supermarkets where you can.

WHY RED MEAT SHOULDN'T BE FEARED

Alongside the vegan craze of recent years, we've seen red meat become the supposed bad guy for all of our society's health issues – obesity, type 2 diabetes, cancer, heart attacks, IBS; you name it, apparently the reason for it all is red meat. Really? First off, how on earth did the human race survive for millennia eating red meat if it's so bad for you? Shouldn't we have all died off thousands of years ago when the cavemen and women were eating meat-only diets? And what about people like the Inuits, who survive primarily on a high-fat diet of meat and fish?[21] And the Maasai Mara tribe in Kenya, who mainly eat roasted meat?[22]

It's a controversial issue, and scientists and researchers have disagreed over the 'is-meat-good-or-bad?' debate for decades. We know, however, that red meat is a really good source of not only protein, but also vitamin B12, folate and heme iron. We also know that obesity wasn't an issue when our diets were less processed and more based on the traditional meat and two veg set-up. I don't believe the problem we have now is people eating simply too much red meat, it's the veg oil, carbs and chemical additives that often come alongside them that are creating our current health catastrophes!

Take a sausage roll. People will say this 'meat product' is bad for you. Yep, I agree, it *is* bad for you. But look at the ingredients list for Tesco's frozen sausage rolls:[23]

Water
Wheat Flour [Wheat Flour, Calcium Carbonate, Iron, Niacin, Thiamin]
Pork Belly (16 per cent)
Palm Oil
Salt
Sage
Caramelised Sugar
White Pepper
Raising Agent (Ammonium Carbonate)
Nutmeg
Sunflower Oil and/or Rapeseed Oil

Hmmm . . . It's not the meat that really is the issue here, is it? Aside from the shocking fact that you're mainly paying for *water* (I mean, what?), it's worth noting that there is only 16 per cent meat. So, although it's labelled as a red-meat product, it doesn't take a genius to work out that it's all the carbs, sugar and inflammatory veg oils that's likely the stuff that does the harm! I don't think we should be blaming meat for the damage that all these other ingredients do.

When looking at food labels and food studies, take it with a pinch of salt . . . (the Celtic sea salt, not table salt, lol).

WHY YOU DON'T NEED TO GO PROTEIN-CRAZY

Do not panic! As I mentioned, you *don't* need to spend a fortune on salmon and steak because it's not about flooding your diet with only protein all day, every day. I'm not asking you to become one of those humourless gym-bunny types popping boiled eggs every five minutes. You want to consume just enough protein – what Dave Asprey, the Bulletproof coffee founder, calls the 'Goldilocks' amount of protein. There are risks attached to eating too much protein, and especially one of our essential amino acids, methionine. It brings both protective effect – such as improved bone health – but can be harmful if consumed in excess, increasing oxidative stress. Yet another of those confusing scientific facts![24]

What we really need to take from this is the idea of balance. It's about having great protein sources, yep, but also getting energy from fat, fibre and a small amount of carbs, too. Personally, I find it really reassuring to know how much good protein is doing me, but that I don't have to go ballistic trying to cram too much into my system. We want to support our bodily functions and make sure we're transporting the right fuel sources to our mitochondria, powering our cells so we can survive and thrive. Giving them a bit of time out with some intermittent fasting, too, so our cells can recycle and get rid of the waste with autophagy. We're not Fred Flintstone, we don't need kilos of meat!

How I've adapted what and how I eat

I am my own experiment, so I'm constantly looking at trying out new approaches to see how they affect me. As I said, I've recently done the carnivore diet for a month, where you only eat meat, eggs and some dairy. I certainly felt absolutely fine on it, but for me it was pretty boring because I am very excited by food and taste, and that's what I missed. I'm a buffet girl, you know? I missed my picky bits! However, I know lots of people who've done brilliantly on it, lost weight, reversed type 2 diabetes, gained more energy, come off anti-depressant and blood-pressure medication, got rid of fibromyalgia and IBS too. It's not for everyone, but could work as an elimination protocol for anyone with gut issues or allergies. You could try it for a couple of weeks and then slowly reintroduce other food into your diet to see how it goes – it's the ultimate elimination diet.

I've been eating good dairy products and high-provenance meat for a few years now, and I'm going to continue on that path. (My plan is to buy one of those huge chest freezers you have in the garage so I can store a whole year's worth of meat prepared by my local farmer! Did you know the meat from one cow and one sheep can support our family of six people and two dogs for a year?) One new thing I'm now introducing is a day's fast once a week – but it's not nil by mouth.

It's something I learned when I stayed at a longevity clinic, the Lanserhof, who had the most brilliant experts there and cutting-edge protocols. They taught me that you can fast with a small amount of fatty calories, which is great for me as my brain needs those fatty calories to get me going every day. By eating a small amount of bone broth, Greek yogurt with MCT oil and some coconut shavings, I'll stay in ketosis and give myself the chance to clear out my cells, because, as we know, fasting encourages autophagy.

The great thing about doing this is the benefits aren't just momentary; for subsequent days afterwards, your insulin sensitivity comes right down, and so it helps with staving off insulin resistance in the longer term. What's more, you reduce inflammation and subsequent risk of disease.

The way I see it, the amount of stress I build up on a daily basis, and the amount of damage I've done to myself in the past, I need this! So every Monday, that's now my plan. Once I get into the swing of things, it'll be totally doable. I really enjoy drinking my bone broth, and with salt and a bit of butter and MCT powder in it as well, it's creamy and much more palatable. It also gives my body the amino acids it needs, so calms my cravings down, and my brain tells me *it's all right, you don't need a croissant, sorry about that*! I'll use my keto monitor – a great piece of easy wearable tech that stays on my arm – to check that I stay in ketosis. Again, this is a type of intermittent fasting, which we've explored throughout this book. It's such a cool protocol for increasing our resilience and living longer.

WHAT TO LOOK FOR IN PROTEIN SUPPLEMENTS

There is a huge market out there for supplements – such as powders, bars and drinks – that promise to supercharge you with protein. However, not all protein supplements are created equal, and first off, of course avoid *anything* that's a UPF, no matter how healthy-looking the label. All those protein bars, snacks and balls that cost a small fortune? Check the ingredients list and I bet you'll want to give them a swerve after you see what's actually *in* them.

You might think protein powders are a safer bet, but all too often they can be highly inflammatory, too. Lots of powders out there are ladened with sugars and sweeteners, like aspartame or sucralose, which can detrimentally impact your health and wreck your gut, completely negating the benefits of having the frigging protein powder in the first place! Many powders also contain artificial colours and flavourings as well as fillers and additives: harmful, unnecessary chemicals that your body will not thank you for. Just take a look at some of the ingredients in one of the market-leading vegan protein powders:

Protein Blend (92 per cent) (Pea Protein, Fava Bean Isolate)
Flavourings
Vegetable Creamer (Sunflower Oil, Natural Flavouring, Antioxidant (DL-Alpha-Tocopherol))
Thickener (Xanthan Gum)
Sweetener (Sucralose)

This is complete junk that will leave you bloated, uncomfortable, inflamed and *craving* carbs after consuming all those sunflower oil, thickeners, additives and chemical sweeteners. So if you want to supplement with a protein powder, make sure it's a decent one, ticking all these boxes:

- complete amino-acid profile
- recognisable ingredients list
- no artificial sweeteners (stevia is OK)
- no additives, GMOs or preservatives
- where your protein comes from (its provenance) – was it grown with pesticides?

How protein powder helps my high street palate

I am a complete and utter child of the 1980s and will never fully get rid of my high-street palate that craves cheap chocolate! But thank God I'm able to mitigate this now with decent protein powders that give me that hit without the horrific after-effects. I like to finish my meals off with something sweet, so I'll often have a small vanilla or chocolate protein shake afterwards. (Full disclosure, my WillPowders bone broth-based protein is all we consume at home.) Or it's really handy to drink before you go out for a meal and have to deal with the temptation of the bread basket – or the dessert trolley!

Another couple of good ways to use protein powder is to stir it through some Greek yogurt – you can then either freeze it and use it as an emergency 'ice cream' with some activated nuts for more satiety. Or you can simply stir Greek yogurt through some nuts and eat it straight away if you need a snack and can't wait! It's great for when you're feeling peckish and sitting in front of the telly – it'll stop you reaching for the KitKats, which really is what we're aiming for here, isn't it? That feeling of having pressed pause on your cravings because you feel full and satisfied. *Lovely.*

PROTEIN, COLLAGEN AND OUR SKIN

When we look our best, we feel so much more confident. I strongly believe that it's completely fine to want to look great from the outside, as well as looking after our health from the inside. We shouldn't feel guilty about it! Obviously I do think about my own skin health because it's the first thing I see every day. What I've discovered in recent years is just how closely protein and especially collagen are aligned with skin health, and in ways that I never knew before.

Most of us know by now that collagen is a beauty buzzword because it gives our skin firmness and elasticity. We've already covered just how essential collagen is, and how we have it all over our bodies. As we age, the wrinkles and sagging skin associated with getting older are indications of poor collagen health; we simply make less of it.[25] Of course, there are now numerous ways we can try to restore this lost bounciness with 'tweakments' such as Botox and fillers, and I certainly wasn't immune to this temptation! However, this doesn't always go to plan – and my experience shows you what the risks can be . . .

My journey with fillers

When I was thirty-nine, I had fillers put in. Of course, there's no coincidence that it was just as I was about to turn forty – I was having a bit of a wobble. I was also training for the London Marathon and had lost a bit of volume in my face. I asked the clinician what I needed to do now I was about to turn forty, and she said, 'Well, you don't want that runner's face, do you? You need more structure.' She advised cheek fillers, and I was like, *hey, fill them up!* That's me all over, really – I take far too many risks, I just wing it and hope for the best. And then what happened? I wrecked the right side of my face!

I had 'temporary' hyaluronic acid fillers, which I was told would dissolve over time. Long story short – they didn't. On one side of my face some old bits of filler had got stuck somewhere, which left my eye looking puffy and swollen as it couldn't drain properly. I was so sick of looking asymmetrical, I decided to get it clinically dissolved using something called *hyalurodinase*. Now, the clinician did warn me that I'd lose a lot of volume this way, but it was still a shock to see how baggy my skin was underneath; my skin had become so artificially stretched with the silly filler over the years that I was left with a long dent. The dissolver also removed my own collagen, making the dent even more pronounced.

HOW TO GET GOOD SKIN WITHOUT FILLER AND BOTOX

After this, I decided that I was going to biohack my way into restoring my lost collagen. Now I'm in my late forties, I can't expect my body to generate the level of collagen it needs by itself, so I'm treating it like a project, and thinking, *OK, this is interesting*, there must be other women out there who put some stuff in their face and ended up looking like One-Eyed Willy from *The Goonies*! I'm turning it from a negative into a positive and attacking it from the inside *and* the outside.

Aesthetic treatments I'm trying out include *polynucleotides*, a type of bio injectable. It uses DNA strands from salmon roe, which contain stem cells, to stimulate your own collagen regrowth. I'm also having some fractional laser treatment on the area underneath my eye, which will do the same, even though it left me looking like I'd been in a proper fight for a few days. But the result should be ending up with smoother skin which won't move about like fillers do. On top of this, I have tried PRP bio filler which is a natural, autologous treatment which uses my own blood to create an injectable gel which smoothes wrinkles and rejuvenates the skin. By the way, I am only treating one eye to try and get my face symmetrical – and weirdly enough, it's the same side as my sarcastic eyebrow. That's karma for you!

It is also worth pointing out that bone health and density are paramount for the skin on your face (and around your body) to hang properly and look taut and full. As we age our skulls shrink, so the more we can do to look after our skulls and boost bone density through supplementation, the more youthful we will look. I mentioned some supplements earlier that I am going to look into, and mouth taping would also help in encouraging nasal breathing that keeps our mouths in the right position.

To be honest, it was a shame I put filler in my face in the first place – I didn't really need it, and it's caused all manner of issues. And I don't use Botox, either – I'm quite happy with my expressions, particularly when I'm having one of my rants!

As well as the above, which I know are pretty costly, I'm trying lots more affordable hacks to restore my collagen from the inside, too – outlined below. Through my research, I've uncovered some amazing information, especially about the role of glycine, one of collagen's amino acids.

WHY GLYCINE IS NATURE'S OZEMPIC

One third of collagen is made up of glycine, and it is absolutely bloody incredible to discover all the roles it plays in our bodies. Firstly, it supports the actual production of collagen – if we don't have enough glycine, we won't make enough collagen, end of. It also converts to glutathione, an anti-oxidant which combats the harmful effects of oxidative stress in our bodies (remember that from earlier?). We use it to produce the muscle-building compound creatine, it prevents inflammation, counteracts the effects of too much methionine (it makes it non-reactive) and can protect our heart from damage, too.[26]

One particular benefit of glycine I find absolutely *fascinating* is that it counteracts excessive sugar intake in the liver by stimulating a hormone called GLP-1.[27] Basically, when we eat foods containing glycine, it triggers this hormone release, which sends the messages to our brain telling us we're full – the satiety response. This is *exactly* what the weight loss drug Ozempic is mimicking! That's the pathway that everyone from Hollywood to Holyhead is attempting to access with pharmaceutical drugs.

If we're taking Ozempic rather than absorbing real glycine through our food, we get the effect without any of the collagen-stimulating benefits; which is why there's the phenomenon of 'Ozempic face', where people look super-thin, very drawn and *very* elderly. There is no need to take this synthetic pathway to get the benefits from glycine. We can get it from our diet.

Peptide Q&A

So what is GLP-1?

GLP-1 stands for glucagon-like peptide 1 and is a peptide hormone which is produced in the gut and released after eating. Once you consume food, GLP-1 is secreted through your intestine and helps to manage the insulin and glucagon response. When it is in good working order, it will let you know when you are full and satiated.

What is a peptide?

Peptides are small chains of amino acids, linked by peptide bonds. They are the building blocks of proteins and perform all sorts of functions in the body. Insulin, for example, is a 51-amino-acid-long peptide hormone and was the first peptide ever to be made in a lab as a medical treatment. Researchers have been working on developing peptide treatments for over a century and Ozempic is the treatment that is currently getting the most attention.

Why isn't Ozempic all it's cracked up to be?

As mentioned above, Ozempic mimics the function of the naturally occurring GLP-1, but unfortunately it comes with some nasty side effects. Lots of people report unpleasant and persistent nausea while using the drug and we see alarming muscle loss. It surprises me that the FDA chose to back this drug when there are others that do the same thing but don't seem to have the same impact on muscle mass, e.g. Retatrutide. (Although let's not forget all of these peptides will cause a rebound when stopped.)

Why are they best avoided for weight loss?

These drugs are invaluable for people with diabetes; however, I wouldn't rely on them if you want to live a long and healthy life. Why disrupt your body's natural processes when you can support them with your lifestyle choices? With some simple biohacks, you can get your metabolism working *for* you, without the need for drugs. Of course I understand that after decades of being told that we should be skinny at all costs, women are turning to Ozempic and Mounjaro, but I hope once we are all more educated about how to hack our metabolism ourselves, we can stop lining the pockets of the pharmaceutical companies that make them and invest in ourselves instead. (FYI, Ozempic and Mounjaro are both made by the same pharmaceutical company, Novo Nordisk, which has a turnover that equals the GDP of Denmark!)[28]

FOUR EASY WAYS TO ELEVATE COLLAGEN FOR GREAT SKIN

1. Eat fatty cuts of meat

For years, we've been told that if we eat meat we should have lean cuts and take the skin off our chicken to reduce the fat intake. However, by doing this we're getting rid of all the glycine, and thus collagen-promoting parts of it, too. The natural glycine also balanced out the methionine which is contained in the lean meat, so nature had already done its job for us! (And really, aren't the fatty cuts the tastier bits too?)

We need to stimulate our GLP-1 satiety hormonal pathway by eating glycine-rich foods, and that means chicken with the skin on. A ribeye steak instead of a fillet. And if you can, organ meats such as in steak and kidney pie (make sure the crust is veg-oil free), or chicken liver pâté. How well we all ate in the past – these were the sorts of things they were eating in this country up until the 1960s and the industrialisation of the food industry. So, there's nothing controversial here, it's just about going back to how previous generations ate!

2. Drink bone broth and other collagen-rich foods

Glycine is also really effective in counteracting a histamine response, which is a major molecule that causes chronic inflammation.[29] As we know, inflammation causes ageing and all manner of other issues such as poor gut health (due to increasing leaky gut) and skin conditions like eczema, acne and psoriasis.[30] By drinking bone broth, which is very collagen and glycine rich, we're helping alleviate that.

As well as the above, other great collagen-rich or promoting foods include:[31]

- Pork-skin snacks, e.g. crackling
- Eggs
- Nuts (activated)
- Bone broth with grass-fed bovine collagen
- Organ meats
- Skin-on chicken
- Lamb and beef stews
- Traditional chicken soup
- Beef jerky
- Gelatine to make into your own sugar-free sweets

3. Reduce glycation by cutting out sugary food

Collagen is negatively impacted by a chemical process in our bodies called *glycation* – and this is stimulated by glucose. Basically, when our blood-sugar levels rise, glycation takes place, which creates the perfectly named *AGEs* (advanced glycation end products). These are sticky compounds which basically tangle up our beautiful, strong net of collagen, making it less elastic. This has a direct effect on how our skin looks, resulting in lack of skin elasticity.[32] We end up with what experts call 'sugar sag', with our skin extra wrinkly and droopy.

Maintaining steady blood-sugar levels can decrease these levels of glycation by 25 per cent in just four months. I know I have been banging on about the danger of elevated blood-sugar levels throughout this whole book, but honestly, if you need any more convincing, this should be it! When you reduce your sugar load, you are going to start seeing better skin, it's as simple as that. So, if you need any more motivation, think of your skin next time you're tempted by that Wispa bar . . .

4. Reduce oxidative stress with less toxic chemicals

The more oxidative stress we put our bodies under, the less collagen we create. Our bodies want to produce it, but we're distracting them with chronic inflammation and the fact they're far too busy putting out all these little fires in our cells. We covered oxidative stress in a deep dive in the first chapter, but not so much the role of collagen. A few years back, I wouldn't necessarily have thought that collagen would help with your anti-oxidant response. But it does; helping us fight off these nasty invaders, so the more we put it under oxidative stress, the less well it works, and so skin ageing is accelerated.

Polluted air is a big factor here, but of course we can't all move to the middle of nowhere! However, we can reduce our oxidative stress load and improve our collagen health by cutting down the amount of toxic chemicals we expose ourselves to, such as pesticides and heavy metals like aluminium.[33] It's in so many of our everyday items, for example:

Nail-polish remover
Anti-perspirant
Perfumes
Bleach and toilet cleaner
Baby powder
Weedkiller
Furniture polish
Oven cleaners[34]

Do your body a favour by reducing the oxidative stress load and shop for toxic-free alternatives, or just don't use some of these products. Who'd have thought that by ditching perfume, we're helping improve our skin health?

Other supplements and skincare ingredients to try for improved skin health:

Silicium/silicon – this is an essential trace element in collagen synthesis and our skin and hair health.[35] An effective daily dose of silica is 200mg.

NAC+ – there is lots of research supporting how effective NAC is in our skin health as it modulates the inflammatory pathways.[36] A recommended daily dose, according to the team at the Wellgevity clinic, is between 900 and 1,800mg, 3–5 days a week. (Unless you have a sulfur sensitivity, in which case halve the dose and frequency.)

Natural vitamin C – a known pre-collagen booster,[37] we can get it from diet or topical skin creams but also supplement with it – 500mg per day is a safe dose. Try and swerve ascorbic acid as it's a synthetic form of vitamin C – acerola extract is a great option.

Tripeptides – these can be found in some anti-ageing skincare products due to their ability to regenerate collagen levels.

Hyaluronic acid – if you're drinking your bone broth, you'll already be getting the fabulous benefits of hyaluronic acid. This acid is a humectant substance which locks in moisture and makes your skin look plumper. Lots of good brands will sell hyaluronic acid serums.

Astaxanthin – which is a potent antioxidant and considered an internal SPF.[38] It also helps the skin turn gold as it is a carotenoid.

MY TOP FIVE EATING-FOR-LONGEVITY TAKEAWAYS

I hope this chapter has given you some brilliant ideas to flip your thinking about what food can do for your healthspan, and easily accessible, delicious protocols to try out. But do you know what? I don't expect life to be perfect. I'm as easily tempted as the next person. I'm not preaching perfection, because I'm just like the rest of us – I have a Chinese at my local restaurant because it makes me feel like I'm in glamorous Hong Kong rather than Clitheroe (although actually, on a summer's day it's a rather gorgeous place to be!). I use chewing gum even though I know it's full of rubbish. I still do it even though I know everything that I do about veg oil, additives and refined carbs. That's what we humans do; we self-sabotage, we're absolutely *gormless* at times!

So, if you have a moment where you decide to 'treat' yourself with a KFC, and feel shit afterwards, do not worry! Just listen to yourself, listen to your body and what it's telling you. You know when you're bloated, you know when you're feeling crap, you know when you've got a food hangover. This is a framework here to support you, through the rest of your life. It's progress, not perfection. Keep going.

1. **Think protein-first, not carb-first**, and plan your meals accordingly.

2. **Reconsider red meat**: it doesn't have to be the baddy, and is a great protein source.

3. **Investigate regenerative farming and soil quality**: know your food chain and get to know your butcher and farms.

4. **Only use quality protein and collagen powders:** don't accidentally introduce UPFs!

5. **Boost vitamin C intake**, to promote collagen production (not ascorbic acid).

FUTUREPROOF PRINCIPLE #4: GET MOVING

All movement begins in the brain, because all movement starts with a decision. It starts with the decision to do something, or not do it. Often, we make these decisions without even consciously realising that we're making them. It's the difference between making a decision to shuffle over to the fridge, bored, to look for a snack, or to pick up our running shoes and put them on (honestly, this is *always* the hardest part of going for a run for me!). Whether we stand on the escalator or take the stairs. Whether we stay indoors at our desk over lunch or take a ten-minute walk out in the sunshine (well, more likely than not grey drizzle, but you know what I mean). This is why I know I'm not addicted: I still have to *force* myself into a run, every . . . bloody . . . day!!

There are literally thousands of movement-based decisions we make every single day, which, over time, all add up. These micro-decisions and subsequent micro-movements are, you may be surprised to know, really *really* important for our longevity and health, and we're going to take a deep dive into them this chapter. But before we go on, I want to reassure you – **this isn't a chapter about why you need to become super-fit, it's a chapter about how we can enjoy freedom of movement.**

It's not about becoming a marathon runner. Not about becoming a hyper-flexible yogi where you can put your foot behind your head. Not about being able to lift mega-heavy weights. (Although, as you'll know by now, improving your muscle strength *is* absolutely something that's vitally important! Don't think I've forgotten that.) Again, we're going to flip the thinking here and focus in on how we can *all* be more mobile, have that fluidity of movement that we took for granted when we were kids, and explore why it's so brilliant for futureproofing us against pain, illness, depression and disease.

WHY WE NEED TO MOVE

We humans are literally designed to move. Over thousands of years, every single part of our bodies has evolved in the most fabulous ways – enabling us to reach up and throw, crouch and sit down, jump and skip, walk forwards, lift and carry objects. This ability we have to regularly move and *do stuff* is literally how we have thrived as a species![1] We're also designed to be upright – our cardiovascular and digestive systems work more effectively when we're standing[2] (which is why back in the old days people went for 'constitutional' walks after big meals ... and also why bedridden people tend to have bowel issues, as they're permanently horizontal).

Despite these amazing, inbuilt physical capacities, over the past couple of hundred years we've innovated ourselves out of needing to do so many of these physical movements. As we've seen earlier in this book, even though advances in modern medicine have kept us alive for longer, we haven't extended healthspan. We get old, immobile, sick and weak. By getting rid of infectious disease and prioritising speed and ease, we've forgotten about one of the most important facts that kept us humans alive and thriving in the first place – and that's the importance of moving, being active and actually *using* our bodies!

HOW CONVENIENT LIVING HAS BECOME INCONVENIENT FOR OUR HEALTH

We're in an age where convenience is prized above all. It's all about what's the easiest, quickest and cheapest. Look, I'm not pretending I don't love a bit of convenience. Much of it is absolutely brilliant and I would hate to go back to a time when we needed to scrub clean our dirty clothes down by a river. (Can you *imagine*? Thank God for washing machines.) As you all know, I also have a tiny, weeny bit of an online shopping habit! However, we now live in a modern world where we don't have to do pretty much *anything* if we don't want to.

We can get in the car instead of walking. We can watch new movies at home rather than go out to the cinema. We don't have to cook dinner, run errands or even go to the supermarket if we decide not to – literally everything we need can be delivered to our front door. We spend our evenings sitting down watching telly, or gaming, or on our phones. Even the way our *toilets* are designed means we don't engage our bodies properly. (Yes! Do not squirm, but we will be looking into loos properly too – we *are* going there!)

When we combine this with the average tech-enabled desk job where we're sitting at our desks in front of screens for hours on end every day, we're headed for a disaster. Our bodies get less and less used to moving, to putting themselves under usual physical stresses that build resilience and stability. That enable natural movement and full mobility. It's not surprising, though, when there could be days where the only proper physical activity we do is shifting the frigging shopping bags from the front door to the fridge.

All this has rapidly changed in very recent times – as recently as the 1970s, only 20 per cent of people were in sedentary jobs,[3] but now it's more than 70 per cent.[4] Tech via our phones and computers means stuff we would have *had* to leave the house to do only ten to fifteen years ago is now easily sorted in seconds. We might not think this matters much, but it really does.

All these changes add up – not walking so much, not lifting a lot and sitting down for hours and hours each day make us increasingly immobile and can lead to horrendous health problems and even early death. Dr Mark Hyman puts it powerfully, explaining: 'There is a great evolutionary mismatch between our current lifestyle and environment and our genes and biology.' Basically, we're not built to thrive in this sluggish routine – spending hours doomscrolling on our phones rather than being 'constantly on the move' like our ancestors.

WHY 'SITTING IS THE NEW SMOKING'

There has been loads of coverage in recent years about the dangers of sitting down too much, and with good reason. There are lots of horrible stats out there on *sedentary living* – which basically just means sitting or lying down, a state of being where we are barely expending any energy.[5] Here are just a few: it can lead to higher risk of type 2 diabetes, heart disease, obesity, depression and anxiety,[6] as well as our old friend insulin resistance – we'll talk about that again in a little bit. Not only that, but the risk of developing some cancers, such as cervical, ovarian and colon, are now scientifically linked to too much sitting.[7] *Bloody hell.*

Overall, if you sit for more than six hours a day, your risk of dying earlier is 37 per cent (for women) or 18 per cent (for men) higher than for people who sit less than three hours a day. Staggeringly, in the UK, we're apparently sitting for an average of nine hours a day.[8] And it isn't balanced out if we exercise, unfortunately – doing a run or HIIT class doesn't mitigate the risks if you still spend hours of your day sitting at your desk or lying on the sofa. And the problem is, we tend to get more sedentary as we age, not less. The less we move, the less we're inclined to move and these bad habits build up – it's a cycle that establishes itself over time.

DEALING WITH THE AGEING STEREOTYPES

When we think about some of the stereotypes around getting older, decreased mobility is certainly up there at the top, isn't it? Being stiff, fragile and frail is literally how ageing is presented to us in so many ways. Road signs that mean 'elderly people' show two hunched-over figures. Adverts promote products to do the physical work for us, like Stannah stairlifts and step-in baths. Honestly, I see these ads and I'm like, *fucking hell, that's only making things worse, isn't it?* Because taking the stairs is brilliant for us and we're being encouraged not to! And what about those step-in baths? Do you just go in and sit there naked and cold waiting for the water to fill up or empty? How awful is that?

I'm in no doubt that many older or disabled people vitally need these things to help them, but it drives me up the wall that this is how *normal* ageing is presented. The narrative of 'this-is-what's-going-to-happen-to-us-all' inevitability. The way it's framed feels as if it's almost designed to make us frailer! But we don't want that – we don't want to be weak and brittle and terrified of falling over, and reliant on a flipping chairlift to get us up the stairs, do we? We don't want to live in fear, we want to live in confidence. We want to be independent and strong, so having freedom of movement really is going to give us the keys to the kingdom. As Dr Gabrielle Lyon puts it, 'Mobility is essential to preserving your own autonomy and ability to do what you enjoy.' That's more like it!

SO, WHY DO WE LOSE MOBILITY AS WE GET OLDER?

There are lots of reasons why we tend to stiffen up and get less mobile with age, which are the downstream effects of all those habits accrued over many, many years. There is (another!) brilliant book out there that I really rate, called *Built to Move*, which clearly explains what happens to our bodies.

Basically, when we sit down for prolonged periods, we rest our body weight on our femurs (thigh bones) in one position, which means their muscles aren't properly engaged. To keep us stable, we compensate by tensing and tightening our backs and legs instead. But many of us have poor posture, so we're compressing our back discs as we tighten them, potentially leading to back pain. Over time, our body gets so used to being in this static position that when we stand up, we feel that *'owwww'* stiffness as it tries to adapt these under-used bones, muscles and tendons into a new stance.

Sitting for long periods also causes our hip flexors to shorten and weakens our glutes as they're not being used properly. This leads to less stability, reduced range of motion and more risk of falls and injuries.[9] The less we move around, the more insulin resistant we become, too – which is why it's so strongly correlated with the ageing process. It's something Dr Benjamin Bikman explores in his book *Why We Get Sick,* and he's unequivocal on how important mobility is; showing research that demonstrates how closely inactivity is related to decreased insulin sensitivity. He explains how just one week of being inactive can increase insulin resistance up to seven times – which is why the cascade of effects after injury and hospitalisation can be so severe.[10] Basically, the less we move our muscles around, the less they respond to insulin because our lack of activity 'hijacks' our inflammation pathways. (Back to inflammation again!)

THE AMAZING LONGEVITY BENEFITS OF MOBILITY

It really all comes back to that 'use it or lose it' adage – because the less we do, the less we feel we can do, the more it hurts and the weaker and less mobile we become. Everything is connected – one thing leads to another. So, it's super-clear: we need to embrace movement and build more activity into our everyday lives. But do not worry, this is easily done. And it's not all doom and gloom, because not only are the negative consequences out there, but so are the positive results that come from increased activity, and they're absolutely bloody fantastic. For example, going from zero exercise to just ninety minutes total each week can reduce your risk of dying from *all causes* by 14 per cent.[11] Basically, people who move more live longer.

Studies have also concluded that physical movement is an essential component in preserving quality of life as it improves mental wellbeing, reduces inflammation and obesity risk, sarcopenia, cardiovascular disease[12] and overall can be a 'more effective and efficient solution' to treating disease than medical intervention.[13] So, not only will we live longer, we'll have a nicer time while we do – extending that precious healthspan that we're all searching for. There really is no doubt about it – by prioritising movement, we prioritise longevity.

Why even our toilets make us less mobile

Brace yourselves – we're getting super-real here and going to talk about going for a poo. Yep, believe it or not, even the way our modern-day loos are constructed means we're reducing our core stability and mobility. Over the hundreds of years since plumbing systems and flushing toilets were invented – and believe me, I am beyond grateful that they were! – in Western countries we've become accustomed to sitting on the toilet with our legs bent at a 90° angle, with our bums completely supported by the seat.

This is all very usual and proper, we think primly, but back in the day we used to squat down to do our business. Every single human being, no matter what their age, would bend down in a deep squat, and in many countries they still do this – whether for going to the loo or for eating, too. This squatting movement uses multiple muscles in our legs, bums, ankles and stomachs, engaging a vital body mobilisation and regenerating cartilage and muscle fibres. One fascinating collaborative study between Chinese and US universities showed that prevalence of arthritic hip pain was 80–90 per cent lower in Chinese people than Americans![14] They concluded that, incredibly, this huge difference was down to squatting being more prevalent in Chinese culture. The elderly Chinese people had moved like this multiple times a day for decades, keeping their muscles and joints well used and fluid, whereas the US participants hadn't – ending up with severe hip pain.

Squatting is actually better for our organs as well. In the usual sitting position, our colon becomes bent, whereas with squatting it straightens out and becomes not only easier to go, but reduces our risk of developing piles and prolapse, too.[15] So, we need to squat more, not less, as we get older. Just remember our joints are designed to bend!

WHY YOU CAN IMPROVE YOUR MOBILITY WITH EASE

Over the years, I've come to love – and depend upon – my exercise, but I am far from perfect when it comes to building in movement throughout my day. I'm guilty of just jumping in the car after a run without cooling down (or warming up, for that matter). I run hunched, and I sleep hunched with my fingers curled tight and usually wake up feeling stiff. I'm often on my phone and I love a Netflix binge as much as the next person. So, although I'm doing OK, I know I have plenty of work still to do! I am constantly seeking out great little tweaks that I can add in to up my mobility and I'll share them in this chapter – everything from easy, free hacks to some of the most incredible new protocols out there.

Our goal is to have that ease of movement, to feel completely comfortable in our bodies the way we used to when we were little. (I clearly remember flinging myself over the six-foot back garden fence to go and play with my friends without even thinking about it!) Remember, we have this wonderful muscle memory and it will kick in when we start to move around more. It's about gaining more stability, more engagement, helping our bodies become more fluid. One of the best descriptions of great mobility that I've come across, thanks to the fabulous Kelly and Juliet Starrett (who wrote *Built to Move*), is that it *allows you to move freely and effortlessly through space and time.*[16] I love the sound of that because it really encapsulates how this is about freedom and ease. How we want to feel loose and supple rather than constrained and stiff.

If you're feeling doubtful right now about your capacity to become more mobile, I get it. (If you suffer with pain, too, we'll cover that.) But if it's about a mental block, you *can* change – it's all about relearning our associations between place and activity: essentially, changing our habits! We are all creatures of habit, which can make it difficult to imagine a different future. But if there's anything I've learned over the past ten years or so, it is that any, and all, habits can be changed. Everything we do in our lives, we once did for the very first time, didn't we? And introducing positive habits will make it easier to keep doing those positive habits (if that doesn't sound too back to front!). Research shows that stronger habits equal greater activity.[17] So we can futureproof ourselves and keep our bodies in the best condition possible – by moving them.

Quick Mobility FAQs

How is mobility different from overall fitness?
As I've mentioned, great mobility isn't the same as having super-human levels of cardio fitness or strength. You can't measure mobility with weights benched or distance run. Instead, it's about *mobilisations*: how well we can move our joints in different positions than the usual ones we tend to stick to (such as sitting in a chair). Mobilisations target our joints, skin, nerve endings, muscles, tendons, brain and breath by taking our bodies through a spectrum of different positions.

OK, but they sound a lot like stretches to me . . .

They're not the same thing. Kelly and Juliet Starrett put it nicely in *Built to Move*, explaining that stretches tend to focus on putting our muscles into a state of 'passive tension' – i.e. holding it in a position. Mobilisations target way more than just one part of our movement system, they engage all types of other tissues and systems and therefore can help with pain issues, too.

What's range of motion?

Many experts in the field use the term 'range of motion' to describe how well (or otherwise) our mobility is working. Range of motion means the extent (or range) of movement you can move your body around a particular joint, such as the ankles, wrists, hips, knees, etc.

Range of motion will be different for all of us. There are some naturally super-flexible people who will have a wide range of motion, and some others who couldn't touch their toes if you put a fifty-quid note on the floor! But don't take your range of motion as a reason not to implement mobilisations. Even the most bendy people will stiffen up as they get older without regular practice, and even the most inflexible of us can make improvements.

Right, so how can I see how good (or not) my mobility is?

Here are a few easy ways you can test various aspects of your mobility from home. The good news is, none of them are super-scary, or difficult to understand. Wherever you're at with each one, do not fret! You will – and can – improve. These are simply ways to gauge your approximate

161

level of mobility, and mean you can regularly check in with yourself, and apply some tweaks if needed.

FIVE MOBILITY CHECKS YOU CAN TRY RIGHT NOW

The squat test

- From a standing position, gently squat down to see if you can rest your bottom on the back of your calves. Keep your heels on the ground while you do so, and slowly unbend your knees to standing again
  - *If your heels pop up*: you might have limited ankle mobility.
  - *If you can't squat down all the way*: you may have hip and/or knee mobility issues.[18]

The sit-and-get-up test

- Stand up and put one foot in front of the other. See if you can sit down on to the floor into a cross-legged position without holding on to anything for balance (channelling those primary-school assembly vibes!). Now, see if you can get back up off the floor, without using your hands or knees or anything else to prop you up.
  - *If you needed to brace yourself, or balance with a hand/knee*: you may need to work on your hip mobility and/or balance.

The stretching-out test

- Lie down on the floor with plenty of room around you. Start with your arms down by your side and gradually bring them up and over your head to touch the surface behind you. Bring them slowly back to your sides.
  - *If your back arches a lot, or if one/both arms are not able to touch the surface:* you might need to improve your shoulder mobility.

The sofa test (borrowed from Built to Move)

- Stand in front of your sofa, facing towards the TV. Bend your right leg and tuck it into the part of the sofa where the seat and back meet. Keep your left foot on the floor, resting the shin against the sofa, but bend your left knee. Now squeeze your bottom while breathing slowly. Swap sides and do it again.
  - *If you struggle to get into position, can't squeeze your glutes or do this on one side:* you may have issues with your hip range of motion and have tightness in this area.

The standing-on-one-leg test

- Stand with bare feet on an even surface. Bend and raise one leg off the floor, in whatever way feels comfortable to you (in front or behind you). Now, close your eyes and start counting! Try to reach twenty. See how long you can stay balanced before you need to reach for a surface or put your foot down. Swap sides and try again.
  - *If you needed to touch the floor a few times, or couldn't count beyond a few numbers:* you may need

to focus on your balance through receptors in your muscles and fascia (more on that soon!).

FOURTEEN WAYS TO IMPROVE YOUR MOBILITY EVERY DAY

Just by googling 'mobility exercises' you'll come across a million and one ways you can improve your range of motion, flexor strength, get better balance and practise all sorts of mobilisations involving resistance bands, etc. I'm not here to tell you *not* to do these – far from it! There are some excellent ideas out there from experienced and qualified people. However, I'm all about building these new protocols into everyday life. How realistic is it that I'm going to do these along with all the other stuff I've got to cope with on a daily basis, like job, kids, husband, dogs, exercising and that last-minute school meeting I've got to dash to when it's pissing down with rain outside? *That's* the sort of protocol I'm interested in!

With this in mind, I've created some simple hacks for you to apply to improve your mobility during your everyday – whether at home or at work. For the work ones, it doesn't matter if you're working from home or in a shared office, you can still do them. With the home hacks, I've divided them up into the rooms you can practise them in. So, it doesn't matter whether you're boiling the kettle, settling in for a *MAFS* marathon in bed (it can't be just me, surely?), or even going to the loo, believe it or not, we can build in tiny yet effective mobilisations everywhere – not just at the gym! It's all those small considerations and little things you can change which will make a big difference.

Five hacks for better mobility at work

Move your bin

I love this tip because it is just so easy and you can do it in seconds: move your bin. That's it! Most of us have our office bins just under our desk, or within chucking distance. If you WFH, take it into another room, or if you're in an office, move it as far away as you possibly can without annoying somebody in HR. There you go – you've instantly given yourself a few more opportunities to get up out of your chair and go for a tiny walk. I'd also add to this, drink plenty . . . and use the loo one floor down if possible. Remember, even walking to use the facilities counts!

Take phone calls standing up

Did you know we have these amazing things now called 'mobile phones', which don't have wires or plugs? They mean we can stand, walk or even run while talking to somebody? It's a miracle! Yes, of course I'm being very, very sarcastic here, but honestly, why on earth do so many of us still insist on sitting down when we chat on the phone, like it's still 1993 and we have to stay in the hallway with the cord wrapped around our hands? It's *nuts*. Next time you take a phone call – or even a video call via your phone – stand up and stroll around while you chat. It'll become a learned habit in no time. I actually do it automatically as it helps my ADHD brain think more coherently.

Don't eat lunch at your desk

This is another modern-day habit that we never used to have, but over the past couple of decades it's become completely normalised to barely leave our desks, even for lunch. Whether you bring in your own home-made stuff, or pop out for a Pret (steering clear of the ham and cheese croissants!), more and more of us simply bring our food back and eat it in front of our screens while continuing to tap away. Do not do this! Eat that lunch and then get out for a walk – even better, take your lunch out to eat elsewhere. (Remember, sunglasses off to get proper blue light from the sun to boost your mood.)

Even if you work somewhere without much green space, just getting out for a short walk along the pavement to play count-the-vape-shops will bring really powerful benefits. Walking for just twenty minutes a day can reduce our risks of developing heart disease, dementia, cancer and diabetes by up to 40 per cent. It might not seem like the most high-octane type of exercise, but it makes a big difference – building in that walking time will help contribute towards a proven longevity protocol. As Dr Mark Hyman says, exercise and movement are 'one intervention that can help reverse most of the hallmarks of ageing'.

Exercises to do in your chair

Standing desks have become super-fashionable in recent times as they make it so much easier to reduce your sitting time. If you can afford it, then it might be worth investing in one – or seeing if your employer will – but even if they're out of your price range, do not fret! You can make seated desk work better for you.

Set an alarm on your phone for once an hour or so, and every time it goes off, do these three movements[19] a few times – none of which demand that you leave your chair:

- *Gunslinger*: lace your fingers together with the index fingers stuck out together like a gun. Now straighten out both your arms and gently dip your head down. Hold for ten seconds, bring arms back to your chest, and repeat.

- *Neck tilt*: Rest one hand on top of your head and tilt it carefully on to one side. Hold for ten seconds, bring it back to the centre and swap hands. Repeat.
- *Chest opener*: Put your arms behind you, lace fingers together and stretch out. Hold for ten seconds, rest and repeat. (Don't forget to breathe!)

Get better balance on your commute

This is a fabulous little tip if you have to use public transport to get to work. Instead of getting into the daily bunfight for a seat on the bus/train/tube, stand up instead – but try not to hold on to anything. Now, there's a challenge! This can be easier said than done, especially with some lunatic bus drivers, but just the action of trying to stay upright will mean you engage your core and your legs in all sorts of ways you wouldn't otherwise, improving your balance and overall strength.[20]

Nine hacks for better mobility at home

In the lounge

Get down on the floor

We all love our cosy sofas, but remember the sit-and-rise test? Research shows that there is a super-clear connection between improved longevity and ability to get up and down from the floor.[21] One simple way to start building this into our everyday is by sitting on the floor rather than the sofa in the living room. Sitting on the floor has been shown to benefit posture, flexibility and strength, and can help with pain reduction in the neck, shoulders and back, going some way to mitigate the horrendous effects we've seen from our overly sedentary lifestyles.[22]

Try sitting either with legs folded underneath you, crossed in front or with them stretched out in front. You can use the front of the sofa as a back rest – and *voilà*, an easy way to improve longevity while you're watching trash TV!

Fidget!

I was forever being told to stop fidgeting when I was younger, but it looks as if I was on to something without realising! The micromovements involved in fidgeting, whether that's bouncing feet, jiggling legs, tapping fingers, *whatever*, have now been scientifically proven to improve mobility and longevity. It sounds bonkers, doesn't it, but by fidgeting we expend more energy, engage muscles and can even reduce our stress levels.[23] So feel free to move about, even when you're sitting down – I only wish I could have told my old teacher that I was *in fact* practising a longevity protocol, not just being an annoying eleven-year-old. The only caveat to this is that if you think your fidgeting is a sign of stress, you should investigate ways to soothe your nervous system such as breathing techniques and enhancing your sleep.

In the kitchen

One-leg balance practice

Make the time while you're boiling your kettle count. Rather than those pointless tips to 'lift a can of beans to improve your muscles!' (which we've already seen is a complete waste of time), you can make the most of those few minutes by improving your balance instead – a vital component of longevity. There's a clear link between not being able to stand on one leg for ten seconds and a much higher risk of dying from all causes sooner[24] – apparently it is one of the clearest, simplest scientifically backed indicators out there.

So, while you're waiting to make a cuppa, practise standing on one leg with your eyes shut and count. Just don't attempt to pour out the boiling water before opening your eyes!

Stand before you eat

We've now seen how important it is to reduce our sitting time, but what's amazing is *when* that can have the strongest effects. A fascinating study found that sitting for two hours before a meal actually increased your blood-glucose response to that meal – increasing your risk of insulin resistance.[25] So rather than feeling we need to eat while standing up, it's the bit before that's more important.

In the bedroom

Move the telly

I usually end up watching more telly in our bedroom than the living room – mainly because the dogs have all the space downstairs, and my boys are busy 'benching' in their home gym! There's nothing I enjoy more than relaxing in for a three-hour *MAFS*, *Bridgerton*, *Love is Blind*, or any other marshmallow-brain TV marathon. It's my happy place. However, the TV is to the left of the room, and I sleep on the other side of the bed. This means that I spend hours watching telly with my body rotated at an angle and my head tilted to one side – misaligning my body and so exacerbating any stiffness in my neck and shoulders.

If this is you, like me, simply think about moving this around. Can you move the TV so it's not at an angle? Or can you swap sides of the bed so you're more front-on? Or sit yourself in a completely different position? If you watch TV on an iPad, make sure it's at a good height for your neck and head. Try to be as evenly aligned as your room allows.

By the way, I know I should not have a TV in my bedroom, but one day I'll have a nice quiet place downstairs for just me and the dogs once we get that extension built! (Don't hold your breath.)

Unclench your hands

A physio recently shared this brilliant little hack with me, which really helps with releasing muscle and tendon tension. When you lie down in bed and settle down to go to sleep, notice how you position yourself. Many of us – myself included – naturally default to a side sleeping position where we pull our hands close into our chests, and tightly bunch our fingers into a fist, which automatically tightens our shoulders. Just try it tonight you will see what I mean. His advice was simple: unclench your hands! Release your fingers from their tight fist and let them go, into whatever relaxed place they naturally find. Do this and you'll realise you immediately let go of tension around your upper body, and especially your neck.

Put your socks on standing up

Another brilliant tip I found in *Built to Move* is to try to stay standing when you put your socks on in the morning. It's not as easy as some of the other hacks, but is fabulous for improving your balance and core strength. Put your socks down on the floor and reach down to put them on one by one, bending and raising each leg as you do so. Try not to hold on to anything for support! Even if you can't do it at first, keep trying. Just the daily repetitive motion of this will improve your mobility over time.

In the bathroom

Put a footstool in the loo

Squatting while we go to the loo is so much better for us all round,[26] but the last thing I would suggest is getting rid of our lovely, hygienic toilets (I'm not a maniac!). Instead, you can get the benefits of a more squatted position by putting a small footstool next to your loo. Next time you need to go to the loo, rest your feet on it instead of the floor, which will lift your legs and realign your colon.

There are specialist toilet footstools out there, but quite honestly you don't need to bother. You can pick up a super-cheap toddler step from somewhere like IKEA; or if you're my age or older, you probably remember the mania for step aerobics back in the 1990s. If so, it could be time to get the old stepper out of the attic – and finally put it to some decent use!

In the garden

Skip!!

You might think skipping is only for kids in the playground, but it's actually an incredible benchmark test for all sorts of longevity hallmarks, such as co-ordination, motor skills and nerve function, not to mention the health of our fascia – much, much more on fascia below. It improves muscle mass and bone mineral density as well, over time reducing your risk of falls and injury.[27]

You don't even need to use a skipping rope, just the sort of skipping where you lift your knees up one at a time and bounce around is good enough. Don't worry about looking daft. If you have a back garden, do it there! It'll put a smile on your face, too. I actually do a forward skip on the treadmill ... see if you can still do this!

DEALING WITH PAIN

Now, I understand if you've been reading this chapter thinking, *Well, this is all well and good in theory, but I can't do these mobilisations because I have dodgy knees/a gammy back/frozen shoulder, etc.* . . . If you're struggling with pain and finding it's severely impacting your life and preventing you doing what you want, I sympathise. It's utterly crap.

Pain is everywhere, affecting millions of us in various different ways, although back pain and joint pain are two of the most commonly cited types in the UK. What's shocking is just how prevalent physical pain is – stats show that more than a third of women (38 per cent) and nearly a third of men (30 per cent) cope with chronic (persistent) pain. This only increases as we age, with around 53 per cent of over-seventy-fives reporting chronic pain.[28]

We've spoken about pain throughout this book as a hallmark of ageing, and all the protocols, tips and advice covered so far are all designed to help reduce our risk of developing pain-related conditions throughout our life. Cutting down on inflammation, building stronger muscles, eating more protein and getting more mobile will all help build resilience here. But of course, lots of us will already be dealing with pain in various horrible forms!

I'm no stranger to this – I have regular pain in my back and neck. For the past twelve months I have been suffering from a weird frozen shoulder that seems, for a lot of women (myself included), to be linked to perimenopause. I have spent a fortune on massages, red-light therapy, ice therapy and chiropractor appointments. However, what has really helped has been upping my oestrogen-supporting supplements. My favourite ingredients are black cohosh, wild yam and Kudzu flower, which I believe have boosted my body's natural production of anti-inflammatory oestrogen. No more massages needed; and if that hadn't worked, I would have started looking for other options and most likely started investigating BPC-157, a peptide which is not yet FDA approved, but in time looks like it could be a promising treatment for musculoskeletal injuries.

There isn't much I wouldn't try, to be honest, because this shoulder was stopping me from doing upper-body exercises and therefore reducing muscle mass and tone (particularly on the backs of my arms), and impeding my immune system, thus making me more vulnerable to infection and subsequently lowering my self-esteem.

WHY AND HOW WE FEEL PAIN

What I've found massively inspiring (and helpful) over these past few years is discovering just how pain works – where it comes from and how and why we experience it. The actual sensation of pain is a series of messages between our brain and the site of the pain – no matter where that is. Our bodies are incredibly sophisticated machines, and wherever there is nerve damage it causes electrical signals to be sent to our spinal cord (the vagus nerve). At this point those messages become chemical – neurotransmitters – and are sent to our consciousness. It's all part of our nervous system!

An absolutely spot-on explanation from Kelly and Juliet Starrett is that *pain is a request for change*. When we feel pain, our body is signalling that something is wrong, and the brain interprets this as a threat. It doesn't always mean that we have a horrendous injury – it can be down to all sorts of reasons like inflammation, low salt, poor sleep, not moving enough, dropping sex hormones (more on this later); indeed, any of those crappy habits we've developed through our convenience-first modern lifestyle.

APPROACHING PAIN DIFFERENTLY TO IMPROVE OUR MOBILITY

It's important to remember that pain is registered in the brain, which is why our nervous system is so important here – and we're going to explore that very soon. What's more, when a body part hurts, the root causes of that pain very often lie elsewhere; the pain is just the downstream effects of other problems going on. Knee pain could be an issue of connective fascial tissue (more on fascia in a mo), an aching back could be down to stiff quads. Our bodies are completely connected, as we've seen already, so addressing the *root causes* of pain is vital, rather than just chucking paracetamol (or something stronger and more addictive) down our throats for the rest of our days.

Look, I'm not claiming that I can eliminate anyone's pain – but again, I just want to flip the thinking about how we treat pain. Sales of over-the-counter pain medication reached £749 million in the UK in 2023[29] and around 10 million people suffer daily with pain that negatively impacts their life.[30] This isn't progress, this isn't enjoying life and thriving, it's just existing in addiction, and damaging the liver and gut, thus making us vulnerable to disease due to a weaker immune system. And unfortunately, pain medication doesn't solve the problem, it's just a temporary fix. To round up this chapter, we're going to explore two different ways of improving our bodily pain and boosting mobility in the process: by targeting our fascia and our nervous system.

FLIPPING THE THINKING #1: FANTASTIC FASCIA

Fascia is probably one of the most underrated areas of our body's biology. We are literally full of the stuff, but when was the last time you heard anyone talk about it? Luckily, it's becoming more and more widely understood – what it is, what it does, how it impacts our mobility and also its relationship to pain. (I have become borderline obsessed with a really pioneering woman in the States called Ashley Black, who is all about fascia care and invented a tool that I'm currently using – more shortly!)

But first. *What on earth is fascia?* I hear you ask. Basically, fascia is a type of stretchy, sticky connective tissue that we have all around our body.[31] It's wrapped around all our vital organs, muscles, tendons and cells, holding them in place, and is a living, strong thing full of multiple layers. Think of it as sheets of soft tissue that provide a flexible yet robust framework that enables our bodies to function, keeping our muscles, ligaments, bones, organs and tissues separate and stable.[32]

Fascia is mainly made up of our old friend collagen and there are a few different types:

- Superficial – found immediately under the skin
- Deep – around our bones, muscles, nerves and blood vessels

- Visceral – surrounding our organs
- Paretial – lining our bodily cavities[33]

Is fascia, not fat, behind cellulite?
One mega-interesting school of thought suggests that fascia could be behind what we've come to call cellulite: when skin appears lumpy and puckered, usually around women's thighs and bottoms. I myself have had cellulite since I was fourteen. I've been big and small, but it doesn't matter, I've always had it. The thing about so-called cellulite is that for years we've been told it's down to fat, whereas the fact is we will all know skinny people with cellulite, and larger people who don't have any! So that has never made any bloody sense to me *at all*.

However, what does make a lot more sense is the idea that it's the health of our superficial fascia that's more important, rather than how much weight we carry. Although not all experts agree on what causes cellulite, one study suggested it was down to a weakness in the superficial fascia, creating a dimpled effect as some parts of the skin are 'pulled down' and fat cells collect between the gaps in connective bands, giving that orange-peel appearance.[34]

The link between fascia, movement and pain

Healthy fascia is essential for keeping us supple and mobile, but its condition can drastically change in either direction: it can become both too loose or too tight. For example, during pregnancy, superficial fascia becomes even more super-stretchy than usual, and even tears on occasion (such as when the abdominal muscles separate, or somewhere else more sensitive . . .). Naturally, fascia can be totally disrupted during weight gain and loss and doesn't always knit back together properly – this is why our skin droops if we've lost a lot of weight.

On the other hand, when our fascia is tense and constricted it can cause pain and health issues. Deep fascia contains pain receptors,[35] and when it tightens up (often due to inflammation or trauma), those receptors spark into action, causing fascia pain. Often when we feel like our muscles are aching, or feel tight 'muscle knots', it's not that, it's actually something called *fascial adhesion*! A good rule of thumb to tell the difference is that muscle pain feels worse when we move it around, fascial pain feels better.[36] *Fascinating.* And inactivity built up over the years can lead to our fascia becoming tighter and less elastic. Yet another example of *use it or lose it.*

There are lots of conditions that are linked specifically to fascia, such as plantar fasciitis – pain and stiffness in the heel – and fibromyalgia.[37] I've heard from a lot of my followers who struggle with fibromyalgia, which is often just dismissed as non-specific muscle pain. Fibromyalgia, however, is increasingly being seen as a result of problems in the fascia. One study showed that fascial inflammation can lead to the increased sensitivity and widespread pain seen in fibromyalgia.[38] All this shows us how fascia plays such a key role in musculoskeletal health, and the fact we have disregarded fascia for so many years is rather bonkers, in my opinion . . .

What I'm doing to look after my fascia

Keeping our fascia healthy is so important, then, for reducing pain and improving our overall mobility. If you're tight somewhere, and your movement is limited, it's definitely worth trying to improve your fascial health. However, it's not something we can fix by doing more sit-ups and squats! We need to treat the fascia itself to help it become more open and supple. Open fascia is said to promote tissue healing because it increases blood flow, leading to improved collagen and better mobility.

There is so much you can do to promote healthy fascia. The first place to look is Chinese medicine. Practitioners use a variety of methods including cupping, gua sha and massage. Currently, I'm using a little piece of kit called a Fascia Blaster to promote healthy fascia. The blaster itself looks a bit like a dimpled plastic stick with spikes (also plastic! Do not worry!) that you rub up and down along your skin. Some women have reported bruising when using the blaster. My advice is to go lightly and let the area loosen up. Much like exercise, we feel it if we go too hard, too quickly. Easy does it – use common sense and be gentle. Chances are you have never treated the fascia, so little and often is key.

I've done an n-of-1 experiment on myself with one leg being fascia blasted (right leg) and my left leg untreated. I've uploaded a picture on Instagram and the result around my calf is quite incredible! I didn't realise you can have non-dimpled cellulite around the ankles and mid-calf! I just have to do the other one now, which will take about two months. There's a smaller blaster for the face, which I'm using to improve blood flow there and tighten up my jaw line.

Over time you will get to know which parts of your fascia are congested and which parts are healthy. You can then tailor your treatments to those areas. With consistency, fascia can remodel over a thirty- to ninety-day period. This technique is now a really important protocol for me to keep my skin glowing and relieve wrinkles without resorting to Botox . . .

FLIPPING THE THINKING # 2:
NEURAL RESET THERAPY

Right! Remember how pain is registered in the brain? But how most pain treatments try to fix the problem with medication (masking the symptoms) or physio/massage (only targeting the symptom, not the root cause)? There is a very exciting field out there called *neural reset therapy* or sometimes *neuro reset technique* (NRT in both cases, conveniently!), which can treat pain – amongst many other issues – by accessing the nervous system.

Explaining NRT can get tricky, and I am far from a trained practitioner, but here goes. NRT treats the body by accessing the messaging going on between the brain and the muscle function. Symptoms like a bad back or a sore knee are symptoms of a nervous-system problem where you can't recruit your muscles well enough, and there is an 'immature' connection between the brain and that area. NRT aims to reset this by accessing the vagus nerve, a key link in how our brain processes pain, part of our parasympathetic (rest and digest) nervous system. Our nervous system has been described by Jessica Maguire, author of *The Nervous System Reset* as 'a series of networks gathering and sending information', with our brain working as a sort of 'head office', processing the information sent from different sources around our body, which are often dysregulated.

I have seen an NRT therapist called Simon Frost in London for a few different issues, like a flared ribcage and my shoulder which I spoke about earlier. He's been absolutely brilliant for both me and helping my son Jude with his posture. Rather than spend a fortune and hours and hours on physio, I've used NRT and it's been fantastic in waking these muscles up and improving my mobility and posture. He has also advised I do some Callanetics to support my new posture.

How does NRT work?

Simon studied and worked in various different fields like body work, neuromuscular therapy and PT for many years but became disillusioned when he saw that the traditional treatments weren't providing a long term solution for his clients' problems. 'Often there was the same outcome,' he says to me, which was that many people's issues would come back! So, he developed NRT and explains his approach as 'teaching the brain and nervous system about the physical body so they are able to operate the body effectively and non-consciously'. He practices by stimulating the nervous system through a process of sensory biasing and nervous system strengthening, seeing where there are areas of weakness, and then treating those pathways. Individual treatment depends on the area you're treating, but overall, NRT 'improves the capacity of your nervous system, making it function efficiently and increasing resilience to any stresses'. Simply resetting your posture into optimal alignment can have a huge impact both up and downstream, enhancing wellbeing.

This might sound a bit woo-woo if you've not heard of it before, but Simon Frost's NRT is growing and growing as a field of focus – I really believe it is the future. 'We need to look at what's triggering the symptom and what we can do about it, rather than just give you a pill or a massage every week and you have to just cope with it,' says Simon. 'I'd like people to understand how the brain and nervous system is so important to their health. You become what you experience via input (sense), process (brain and CNS) and output (muscles). So if you are suffering with poor health, it is the sum of the experiences that have led you to feel this way. Continuing to experience the world the same way you did before any type of treatment will not transform your health. To transform we must change our wiring and bring new opportunities for our brain and nervous system to receive and experience the world in a different way, a way that helps people become robust for life.'

So! If you're interested in trying out a drug-free, surgery-free and *super* low-intervention (I mean, you literally do not have any recovery time or annoying exercises to do at home) way of treating pain, improving mobility and reducing stress, I recommend Simon Frost's NRT. There are trained practitioners out there that you can find online, and videos to follow yourself to gen up more on this fascinating protocol.

NRT is arguably similar to acupuncture in the way it interacts with the nervous system. Acupuncture is another therapy I really believe in and would recommend if you are dealing with persistent pain and joint problems. Acupuncture, a therapy whereby small needles are inserted into different parts of the body, is a part of traditional Chinese medicine and has been clinically shown to improve nerve-related disorders. It is another great alternative option that means you don't have to take more medications or put yourself through risky surgeries. Worth a try, if you ask me. I find it fascinating that when you are going through IVF they also recommend acupuncture, and when you ask the doctors why they use ancient Chinese medicine when they are implementing the flagship in Western medicine, they literally have no answer and refuse to acknowledge the power in manipulating the flow of energy. They might say it's relaxing, but I know better ways to relax than putting pins in my skin.

My top five mobility-boosting takeaways

What I find so flipping inspiring with biohacking is how seemingly innocuous changes can have huge impacts. That things which seem utterly inconsequential, like moving your bin, adjusting your fingers and jiggling your legs a bit more, can have downstream effects that will boost your longevity and help you live a life with less (or no) pain. This chapter is full of these types of tiny changes with big impacts, so I urge you to tackle as many of them as you can – it's all about fitting in with reality, too. We can all get a bit obsessive about things, can't we (myself included, naturally)? But there is a middle ground where we make positive changes without putting ourselves under crazy pressure all the time. Better mobility is one of those things that is available to *all* of us.

1. **Sit on the floor**. Such an easy way to engage your core muscles, reduce insulin resistance and improve mobility.
2. **Stand up when on the phone**. I mean, mobiles are supposed to be mobile!
3. **Put a footstool next to your loo**, and you'll have a shortcut to the benefits of squatting.
4. **Set an alarm every thirty minutes while working**. Take a quick break and do the seated mobility moves, or take the opportunity to visit the loo that is further away.
5. **Shine the spotlight on fascia**. Invest in some massage time every week.

FUTUREPROOF PRINCIPLE #5: CALM THE F--- DOWN

I am, by nature, rather a stressed-out person. I get so frazzled trying to organise my life, my work and my kids – and with no extended family to lean on locally, when things go wrong they go *very* wrong! Just recently I was in Germany researching this book and got my dates wrong, which meant a hell of a twenty-four hours: I had to change my flights back to the UK, fit in some filming, then an event, then more work commitments . . . And what made it even worse was all the travelling I had to do, which I hate. My crappy, giant, wonky suitcase kept face-planting on the floor of the train over and over again because I pack too much for fear of not being prepared for all kinds of bizarre weather conditions (classic ADHD). I was pouring with sweat, trying to pick up this useless piece of kit. I was unbelievably flustered! All this because my admin skills are on the floor, and always have been.

However, on the flipside, I think in many ways I thrive on a bit of stress. I need that cortisol – the main stress hormone – boost to give me some get-up-and-go, because I don't find motivation in peaceful situations! I tend to zone out and start daydreaming, whereas during a stressful moment, I jump into action. In some ways, I function at my best when there's some sort of crisis going on. It might be the way I'm wired, it might be down to my ADHD (by the way, people with ADHD make very good police officers, paramedics and chefs – basically any job which requires you to function on high alert!). It might have been passed down from my dad who is very similar to me in this way. (However, he's a demon at paperwork and detail; I still need to develop that skill set!) Who knows? I often think we need some of the population to be wired this way to problem-solve in high-stress situations, and others who are good at planning, like our farmers.

DIFFERENTLY WIRED, DIFFERENT STRESSORS

I understand that, to some people, this will sound horrendous. For those people that can be quiet and still for a long time, the people who thrive in yoga classes and enjoy crafting, I imagine the idea of getting a buzz from chaotic situations would be *awful* for them and spark a huge amount of stress. But on the flipside, what chills them out would be an utter endurance test for me, as I'm no good at sitty-downy gentle things. Of course, that's fine – we are all so different. Once again, it comes down to the idea of the 'tribe' that I've chatted about before – that we all bring something different to our collective human tribe, and that's the beauty of our individual personalities and biochemistry.

This is why I find a one-size-fits-all approach to managing stress unhelpful in the extreme. What works for me to blitz my unhealthy stress levels and find enjoyment – things like listening to house music while running in the pouring rain – might not work for somebody else; in fact, it would really stress them out! The important thing is that we all feel stress, but what creates and alleviates our stress can be very different.

NO BOUNDARIES = MORE STRESS

Although some level of stress in our daily lives is natural – and needed – it can easily tip over into dangerous levels that impact our longevity. Yep, stress can actually be the culprit behind life-limiting disease. And it's harder than ever these days to mitigate and balance all the elements in our lives that are, quite frankly, pretty bloody stressful.

So much of this, I believe, is down to the lack of boundaries caused by our hyper-connected state. The natural barriers that used to exist between the different elements of our lives – work was separate from school, which was separate from home, which was separate from our social lives, etc. – have been completely trampled on. They just don't exist any more! We can be dealing with work emails, trying to put out World War III with the kids, admin, checking social media, doing food prep and a hundred other concerns *all at once*. When you think about it, it's crazy we put ourselves through this, but it's actually very, very difficult to instil those 1990s-style boundaries now. Over time, dealing with everything, all at once, just leads to more stress. I mean, of course it frigging does!

A STRESSED-OUT NATION

There are some shocking stats out there about just how stressed we Brits are these days. Almost three-quarters of adults in the UK say they have felt overwhelmed or unable to cope at points,[1] and a fifth of adults have taken time off work due to suffering with stress. In a global study on different countries' stress levels, the UK ranked joint highest (along with South Africa).[2] It's getting so bad that the head of a mental health charity has warned that we risk becoming a 'burnt-out nation'.[3] Not only is this bad for the state of our NHS – stress, anxiety and depression has now overtaken musculoskeletal pain to be the number one cause of sick leave in the UK[4] – but we'll see later just how detrimental it can be to our healthspan, too.

In this chapter, then, we're going to take a deep dive into stress: how it works from a hormonal perspective, the downstream effects on the body and the brain, and how excess stress is now understood as a direct cause of multiple conditions – not just for issues such as depression and anxiety, but things like insulin resistance, weaker bones, depleted muscle mass and even weight gain. (Flipping heck.)

But do not fret, we are going to flip the thinking yet again. Rather than immediately reaching for anti-depressants, anti-anxiety meds or 'Hey, just relax, OK?' platitudes (because you know what, that is the *last* thing I want to hear when I'm in a high-stress state!), I'll share some really actionable, easy, everyday tips with you that won't feel like just another chore on your never-ending to-do list. We'll be able to deal with stress better when it arrives, and in many cases, get ahead of it before it causes most harm – all without spending thousands of pounds on going to pricey retreats to '*om*' ourselves into a relaxed state. Because we want to futureproof ourselves against damaging stress while living in the real world, don't we?

How stress works in the body and brain

First things first: stress is vital for our survival. We have evolved to have a stress response, so there's no point in trying to eliminate it entirely – we need it. Just like all those hormones and bodily functions that have developed over millennia, it's always a far more nuanced picture than stress = bad. (A bit like the whole cholesterol mixed messaging, but there you go.) So, first up, we need to understand where that stress response comes from and what it's doing.

When we feel stress, we're sending emergency signals throughout our brain and body. Although I went into the hormonal step-by-step in my last book (check out the chapter 'Why Am I So Stressed?' in *Hack Your Hormones* for this), it's worth doing a quick recap just so we understand what's going on behind the scenes during those nerve-shredding sensations. And what I find amazing is that stress hits us at different speeds.

The two-speed stress response

Here's what's happening. When we encounter something stressful, whether that's reading a horrible message on our phone, hearing some unexpected bad news or just some dickhead cutting us up in traffic, it all starts in the brain.

The amygdala – the central part of our brain responsible for processing emotions – registers the stress and sparks various neurochemicals into action. (Nice little fun fact – the amygdala is so called because of its almond-like shape – *amygdale* means almond in Greek!)[5]

Imagine a near-miss car accident. Your eyes or ears register the danger, sometimes in the periphery before you even see the full image. This is the autonomic nervous system kicking in to save your life. You literally don't have time to think, you just act!

The amygdala triggers a cascade of stress responses. First, it sends a signal to the hypothalamus – the 'command centre' of our brain.[6] This then triggers our sympathetic nervous system – our *fight or flight* response – sending a hormone to our adrenal glands which essentially demand a burst of energy in order to deal with this stress. These glands then release **adrenaline** (also known as epinephrine) into our bloodstream.

This all happens within *milliseconds*. Really, it's so quick that we feel adrenaline's effects immediately. Our blood pumping stronger, breathing faster, feeling panicked, wired, with hot and cold rushes throughout our whole body? On complete and utter alert? Sounds familiar? Yep, that's our adrenaline being released. It happens before we even see a situation, like jumping out of the way of a car when crossing the road – instinct.

But adrenaline isn't the whole picture. At the same time, the HPA axis swings into action (HPA means hypothalamic-pituitary-adrenal – it's all right, we'll stick to HPA, shall we?), activating a chain reaction of various neurochemicals that will also raise our **cortisol** levels. This is for good reason – cortisol is fabulous at helping us regulate our stress response. It does this by increasing our accessible energy through glucose release, controlling blood pressure, reducing inflammation and increasing our alertness[7] – ensuring we stay revved up and ready to deal with the continued stressor.

What I find absolutely fascinating is that, unlike adrenaline, cortisol levels don't peak immediately. It can take fifteen to twenty minutes for the cortisol response to be felt, so there is a measurable delay. Now this might seem awful – *oh no, more stress hormones on their way* – but I think it's good news, because it gives us a warning. A little bit of time to know that cortisol is on its way, and we will use this to our advantage later on in the chapter. But for now, what we need to know about the speed of our stress response is that:

Adrenaline: immediate
Cortisol: later

WHEN CORTISOL GOES OUT OF WHACK

The process outlined above is our bodies working as they should. After our hypothalamus perceives the stressor has been dealt with by the cortisol release, our body resets to baseline, by switching off the HPA feedback loop. Or rather, it should. A bit like inflammation, stress is OK when it's *acute* – sweeping into action to deal with a one-off problem – but not when it becomes *chronic* – all the frigging time.

Cortisol is our 'master' stress hormone, and, as many of you will already know, we have a natural cortisol boost after we get up in the morning. Our cortisol levels should naturally peak then and gradually decline throughout the rest of the day. Cortisol performs all sorts of amazing functions in our body in addition to stress, such as regulating our blood-sugar levels, sleep–wake cycles, metabolism, inflammation and blood pressure.[8] A bit like I chatted about in the chapter about eating protein, we need a 'Goldilocks' amount of cortisol – just enough.

However! It will not surprise any of you that if these carefully calibrated hormonal levels are disturbed, we're going to feel some pretty horrendous effects. It is possible to have both too much and too little cortisol in the system. (Yes, as ever, things are never simple!) At either end of the cortisol spectrum, you have two diseases: Cushing's disease is too much cortisol in the blood (*hypercortisolism*), whereas Addison's disease is too little cortisol (*hypocortisolism*).

HOW TOO MUCH CORTISOL MAKES US ILL, INSULIN RESISTANT AND OVERWEIGHT . . .

If we are dealing with constant stress, even if it's low-level, we are putting our sensitive nervous and endocrine systems under non-stop pressure. This dysregulates the HPA axis, which can mean we end up with too much cortisol flooding through our system because it doesn't switch off. This is a big problem even if we don't end up with Cushing's disease – excessive cortisol has been linked to increased inflammation (yes, that one again), metabolic-syndrome diseases[9] like type 2 diabetes and cancer, and even degenerative conditions like Alzheimer's.[10]

Too much cortisol can also make us fat, because of insulin resistance. Excess cortisol raises our blood glucose because it's seeking out that energy to help us deal with the stressor – to make our bodies primed and ready for action. Cortisol will literally make glucose out of *anything* we have available, including fats and protein, not just carbohydrates. In these stressful moments, explains Dr Benjamin Bikman in his book *Why We Get Sick*, there is a battle going on in our bodies between insulin and cortisol. Insulin wants to dampen down our blood-sugar levels, and cortisol wants to raise them. However, cortisol is so frigging powerful – remember, it's the 'master' hormone – it *always wins*. The body prioritises cortisol over every other hormone because it keeps us alive.

This is why, over time, too much cortisol leads directly to insulin resistance, which leads to inflammation, which leads to metabolic syndrome, which leads to weight gain. Oh, and what's more, chronically elevated cortisol levels also increase our appetite so we crave sugary, carby foods more – yes, stress-eating is real![11] Sometimes people end up with 'cortisol belly' or 'cortisol face', as when cortisol levels are extremely high, fat can deposit in the face, which leaves people looking puffy, or in the abdomen, which we see as stubborn belly fat.

(Oh, and to add insult to injury, it's not just cortisol. Too much adrenaline can also cause insulin resistance too. A Yale University study gave people an infusion of epinephrine [adrenaline] to see what happened – and in just two hours their insulin sensitivity plummeted by more than 40 per cent.[12] Now, this study is from more than fifty years ago, which shows us just how long we've known that stress is linked to insulin resistance . . . It seems crazy we don't all know about this from a young age!)

. . . BUT TOO LITTLE IS DAMAGING, TOO

Too little cortisol can cause all sorts of problems too – not least impaired immune regulation by reducing the body's control over cytokine production. This leads to excessive pro-inflammatory cytokines being released (such as IL-1, IL-6 and TNF-alpha) and reduced anti-inflammatory cytokines (such as IL-10). The imbalance can cause chronic inflammation, tissue damage and a higher risk of uncontrolled immune responses, such as cytokine storms, making the body more susceptible to infections and autoimmune conditions.

Low cortisol levels can be down to what some experts call 'adrenal fatigue'. Basically, by being in a constant state of chronic stress, your adrenal glands eventually give up, unable to keep up with the amount of cortisol your body is demanding. The HPA axis is thrown completely out of whack, and your cortisol levels fall off a cliff, leading to extreme fatigue, muscle weakness and complete flatlining, not least a higher risk of mortality down to your depleted immunity.[13]

This is what happens when people suffer from *burnout*, which was coined by a psychologist called Herbert Freudenberger, who labelled it 'the high cost of high achievement'. He first wrote about burnout back in the 1970s, but it's just as on the nose today. We're forever reading about high-powered execs, extreme athletes and workaholics suffering with burnout when their high-stress lifestyle completely overwhelms them: it's a very real thing! Japan seems to take pride in this. The Karoshi culture which translates to 'death by overwork' has become a grim reality to many Japanese workers. Campaigns have cropped up to stop the burnout epidemic in the workplace.

Why we can inherit our stress levels

Believe it or not, we can actually *inherit* a certain level of stress. A pioneering neuroscientist called Rachel Yehuda demonstrated that trauma leaves biological traces. She found that pregnant women who lost a partner in the 9/11 terrorist attacks developed PTSD (post-traumatic stress disorder) and had low levels of cortisol. But not only did it affect the women, these low cortisol levels were found in their babies once they were born, too.[14] Coming soon after the same discovery was made in the offspring of Holocaust survivors, this was groundbreaking because it showed epigenetics in action.[15]

Essentially, the parental trauma 'switched on' certain genetic pathways, which was then passed down to their kids – even though those kids hadn't directly experienced the relevant trauma. This is why *generational trauma* is now understood as very real: epigenetics has shown us so. Most of us will have had family members experience trauma in the past; my grandad was on a ship during World War II, but refused to ever talk about it so I'll never know what he went through. The point is, we may have inherited trauma that affects our stress levels, even if we don't know about it. So, all the more reason we need to know *how* to buffer it.

WHY TOO MUCH STRESS ACCELERATES AGEING

I hate to land this on us all, but chronic stress can lead cortisol to rise as we get older and is linked to depleted brain function.[16] One completely fascinating study demonstrated that biological age 'undergoes a rapid increase in response to diverse forms of stress' – showing that stress literally accelerates the ageing process, too.[17] For one reason, too much cortisol causes mitochondrial damage – remember, the mitochondria is the 'engine' of our cells. This activates various ageing pathways, such as shortened telomeres and DNA damage.[18] Yep, those with excess cortisol flooding their system can see their cells start to deteriorate, increased inflammation, and the slow break down of bone density and muscle.

This all sounds pretty awful, doesn't it? Sorry, I'm just the messenger. But the good news is that there are things we can do that will make a significant difference to our overall health and longevity. The same study on biological age and stress also showed that these negative effects are *reversible* – the cellular ageing went back again once the stress was removed. This even 'raises the possibility of age reversal' (very, very big stuff!). Now, this is absolutely brilliant news – yes, stress is a killer, but these ill effects can be reversed. Just like so many things we've covered in this book, it's great to know that it's never too late to change our behaviours and habits and reap the benefits.

MANAGING OUR STRESS RESPONSE

How do I know where my cortisol levels are at?

It is possible to take a cortisol test – either by going to your doctors or ordering one online. They work by measuring the level of cortisol in either your spit, urine or blood and can be useful diagnostic tools for serious conditions like Cushing's or Addison's. However, it is difficult to establish what your optimal cortisol baseline is in the first place, plus there can be issues with testing, too; if you have your blood taken first thing in the morning, when your cortisol is naturally going to be at its highest, or in the evening when it will be lower, then this snapshot isn't going to be the most reliable. Cortisol levels can fluctuate from day to day, even hour to hour, which makes it a tricky beast.

However, you don't necessarily need to take a cortisol test to check if you're stressed (although definitely go and see your doctor to ask for one if you are concerned). We feel the effects of cortisol all over, and it can present in all sorts of different ways in our bodies and brains. Stress doesn't just manifest itself in snapping at your partner or your kids (although TBH, often that's *completely* understandable). If you're having trouble sleeping, struggling with brain fog, a bad tummy, random aches and pains, headaches, eating too much (or even losing your appetite), these can all be related to excessive stress as well.

Although I need a bit of stress to kick-start me, like I said earlier, I find myself feeling burned out just like anyone else. Very often, I need to switch off and reset when I feel too stressed, or if things are just getting to be too much. The other day I was absolutely done in, so I went to bed in the afternoon and let the kids game downstairs. I tried to watch a film on Netflix, but I fell asleep, just like an old fella! I clearly needed that hour and a half's nap.

There are plenty of times, too, when I feel uncomfortably stressed out and lose my temper. I'm not the sort of person who goes into a sulk, I don't hold on to it – I explode and then say sorry afterwards. I get all that frustration out straight away; I'm definitely more of a warrior than a worrier! Like all of us, I don't necessarily need a number on a graph to 'prove' that I'm stressed – I know it and feel it. (However, I do know that my levels are too high – the Lanserhof team told me so and they even prescribed me five minutes of meditation a day to try and dampen it down . . .)

Why so many 'stress relievers' are foe, not friend

When we try and cope with all the stresses that life throws at us, so many of the things we turn to only make things worse – I should know, because that was my relationship with alcohol for years and years. So, I'm not here to judge *at all*, because in fact modern-day society makes it very difficult for us to resist these unhealthy habits. It takes a lot of knowledge and awareness to break away from the usual suspects that are thrown at us by well-meaning friends and family (and not-so-well-meaning advertising!) when we feel stressed out.

I'm thinking about not only booze, but things like cake and biscuits being framed as a de-stressing 'treat'. I passionately believe we need to explore what other options are out there, which are non-addictive in the long term and that have proper, positive effects on our stress levels, leaving us feeling better mentally, physically and emotionally. But first, let's bust some myths, shall we?

Stress myth-buster #1: 'Have a glass of wine to relax'

There is no safe level of alcohol consumption, no matter how many 'red wine is good for you' articles you might read. Sixty per cent of adults in the UK use alcohol as a coping mechanism.[19] However, it is the literal opposite of beneficial for our stress levels. Alcohol is an addictive substance and amongst other things wrecks our gut – killing off our good-bacteria microbiome, which is where serotonin, the happy, cosy hormone is made. You will feel more depleted and more stressed without serotonin – guaranteed. Oh, and what's more, low cholesterol is linked to low serotonin, too, so there's another reason why statins are linked to depression!

(Fun fact – serotonin is released throughout your gut, as high up as the mouth, via gut sensory cells called neuro-pod cells.[20] The finding of these neuro pods has sparked a new field of exploration in sensory neurobiology – that of the gut–brain sensory transduction. In layman's terms, when you have something like cheese on toast or shepherd's pie, as soon as you taste that food the brain immediately feels cosy and safe. When doctors say there is no such thing as serotonin crossing the brain barrier from the gut, throw the phrase 'What about neuro pod sensory transduction?' at them, and tell them to look up the brilliant work of Dr Diego Bohorquez.)

As women get older, too, alcohol has more of a ferocious effect. As hormones drop and fluctuate, tolerance goes down, so the after-effects are worse and worse. And for men *and* women, drinking alcohol will drive up cortisol at the wrong time (not first thing in the morning, when you want it, but throughout the night!), resulting in lack of sleep and no REM in the sleep you *do* get. This also results in the 'beer fear' – that horrible anxiety that comes from a cortisol spike and depleted dopamine levels. Remember: you may get a temporary boost from dopamine with that first glass, but it pushes your baseline level down over time, so you will just feel more depleted and flatline the more you drink.

I clearly remember my awful hangovers in my late twenties, feeling paranoid and with the worst intrusive thoughts ever. I'm certain that I wouldn't be able to handle that now I'm in my mid-forties – one of the gifts of sobriety is never having to experience the come-down terrors again. If you drink, it's worth taking some time off the booze to see how it affects your stress levels. You'll notice a more positive inner monologue after only a few days.

Stress myth-buster #2: 'Eat something sweet as a treat'

We know the equation by now, don't we? Too many sugary foods = blood-glucose spike = insulin resistance = inflammation = all manner of disastrous outcomes, one of which is lower baseline dopamine.[21] Yep, sugar's not just the reason for our poor health, but poor mood, too. Scientists now believe that sugar overconsumption may be directly linked to soaring levels of anxiety and depression across the world.

However, we are constantly surrounded by marketing and advertising that tells us over and over again that eating a bar of chocolate/doughnut/pudding is the easy route to relaxation and feeling good about ourselves – whereas science has now shown us without doubt that it actually will make us feel physiologically horrendous. I know – *fewmin'*! So, of course it's easier said than done, but whatever you can do to swerve the 'a brownie will make me feel better' pathway, do it. Reread Futureproof Principles 1 and 2 for ways to wean yourself off sugary foods and shift your eating habits, as well as the chapter on 'Why Can't I Stop Eating?' in my last book *Hack Your Hormones* for good places to start. I met Mindy Pelz earlier on this year, who explained that we don't get energy from sweets as we age because the brain, particularly the menopausal brain, becomes more insulin resistant and needs more fat for energy, not more carbs.

Stress myth-buster #3: 'Push yourself harder with a long run/ tough workout'

There can be too much of a good thing! Far be it from me to put anyone off exercise, but it is possible to overdo it, and what's intended as a healthy habit can become detrimental. Any exercise will temporarily raise our cortisol levels – although this is *healthy* stress as it teaches the body the right amount of cortisol to release at certain points.

However, massively excessive cortisol release is a biomarker of what's been called 'overtraining syndrome', where the body is overloaded with physical stress.[22] This is usually linked with people doing endurance sports like running marathons, so if you're only just getting yourself down the gym to lift a few weights, don't stop now, because this won't be affecting you.

I love my running – a bit more on that later – but there is no need to go completely bonkers with exercise. There is a middle ground we can all find. More isn't necessarily better.

HOW TO REDUCE STRESS (WITHOUT GETTING STRESSED OUT)

So, what can we do instead? We are bombarded with advice on how to de-stress, which more often than not can feel stressful, can't it? (Oh, the irony.) Because there are a million and one ways to do it – everything from budget-friendly ideas like going for a walk, to something that will cost you thousands of pounds, like going to a fancy wellness retreat in Ibiza (which, quite frankly, would wind me up anyway). If you can't sit still and do a flipping yoga pose while chanting some transcendental meditation, I understand! It's another fucking to-do thing and that can stress you out in itself. I'd also try to compete, and lose, so I'd become resentful – causing more negative thinking.

I have to do something which is super-cheap and super-accessible, so that's what I've kept in mind with this advice section. As I mentioned before, we're all wired differently, thriving at very diverse wavelengths, so feel free to pick and choose what resonates best with you. And if it doesn't work after a couple of weeks, fine, try something else!

However, I think there's something really important that we should always remember: stress will never go away. Life is full of it, and there is only so much we can do. Yes, there are ways we can reduce or minimise certain things, but the most control we will have is over our response to this stress, not the stress itself. I'm not saying we should become super-calm Zen masters (I mean, that's the last thing I am), but that we have a choice in how we respond, not necessarily in what happens to us.

It is guaranteed that all of us will face lots of stress in our lives – everything from tiny stuff to big, horrific, life-changing calamities. So, instead of stressing about stress, let's focus on how we deal with it, buffer it and think about it. Let's flip the thinking with two protocols on managing stress, and then dive into four mini-sections on how to access some scientifically proven stress-busting pathways: light, temperature, connection and downtime.

FLIPPING THE THINKING #1: EMBRACE YOUR NATURAL CORTISOL BOOST

It's all too easy to become obsessed with thinking of cortisol as the enemy – after all, we mainly speak about the negative effects of too much or too little. But let's remember that it does so much for us – giving us that get-up-and-go, regulating our metabolism and overall trying to keep our bodies and brains fuelled with the energy we need.[23] We need cortisol, so let's not make it public enemy number one – it's not vegetable oil, after all! With this in mind, a first great way to manage our stress response is to lean into it. Yes, we're going to welcome in some stress.

Before you think I've completely lost it, I'm talking about working with your natural cortisol boost that happens in the morning. As we've seen, our cortisol spikes shortly after we get up and then gradually declines over the rest of the day, which is how our bodies have evolved to work optimally. So, if you can, pile your most stressful 'things' into the first part of your day. Schedule difficult work meetings for then, tackle the tricky tasks, do the high-energy stuff that requires most attention and focus.

This is how I try to shape my days – I'm much more efficient in the morning naturally and in the afternoon at work I'm more likely to have more informal conversations, less brain-engagement stuff. (Yes, I used to be a night owl when I was partying, but guess what – it was the alcohol in my system giving me a false energy boost and pushing up my cortisol at the wrong time of day. Since quitting alcohol I've discovered I'm a proper morning lark!)

Of course, I know life often doesn't work like that. We can't always schedule our lives to fit around our hormonal balance, more's the pity. If I've got to do something big, like give a talk or have an important work meeting later on in the day, I'll artificially boost my stress hormones by taking nootropics – supplements that help our brain response and enhance brain performance.[24] When I need to, I'll break out some L-theanine, combined with some caffeine, which gives me about forty minutes of hyperfocus to sort out whatever needs sorting. Whenever I do this, I do feel the ill-effects come the weekend, though, which is when I need to do a proper rest and reset – take a read of the 'Downtime' section for how . . .

FLIPPING THE THINKING #2: GET AHEAD OF YOUR STRESS WITH A FIVE-SECOND HACK

Remember that hormonal delay we learned about at the start of the chapter? That adrenaline races through our system immediately, but that we have a fifteen-minute window before the cortisol kicks in? We're going to use this two-speed stress response to our advantage! We can calm down our cortisol using something called the *physiological sigh*.

Say you've had a shock – a near miss in the car, or just received a shitty work email or school letter – yes, about your little darling! You know your system has registered it because you've felt that rush of uncontrollable adrenaline and utter panic. Now, before you write back a mardy, furious response (I've been there, done that myself), you can take five seconds to buffer the cortisol that's on its way, and in the process become more resilient.

You simply do a quick double inhale – a bit like how crying children look, where they almost 'hiccup' their breath in naturally. Yep, we want to do that, like a sobbing toddler! Breathe in quickly through your mouth or nose twice – the first one up to three quarters of your lung capacity, the second one up to full capacity, then breathe out slowly. And repeat.

The reason it works, Dr Andrew Huberman has explained, is that it 'offloads a lot of carbon dioxide all at once' and increases oxygen to our brain.[25] What's more, this activates our parasympathetic nervous system[26] – our rest-and-digest state – which offsets the fight-or-flight sympathetic nervous response which has been kicked off by the stress. It is incredible to realise that little kids do this completely automatically at the end of a crying fit (and so do we, if we're having a good old sob). By the way, tears are full of cortisol, which is why crying, even with frustration/rage/PMT, is a fabulous de-stressor, too![27]

The physiological sigh is a super-simple, completely free way to reduce stress within five seconds. Do a double inhalation twice or three times (if it's a biggie on the stress front!) and it will lower your cortisol very quickly. Since I've started doing this, it's made me wonder if this is why many of us lean into smoking cigarettes or vapes as a de-stressing technique, because it mimics that sucking in and breathing out mechanism. However, you can get the same effects for free and without any of the horrendous health risks, just by doing this breathing technique.

Try a double inhalation next time something stressful comes at you, and you'll feel more resilient, less panicky and calmer, because you've buffered your stress response brilliantly.

FOLLOW THE FOUR DE-STRESSING PATHWAYS:

1. Light

Getting ourselves into sunlight is pretty much the best free mood boost out there. It's something that we humans have known inherently for millennia, and is why we evolved to be out and about in the daytime rather than at night, but now science can show us exactly why this is. Light is the greatest signal for sparking our bodies' circadian rhythm – our sleep–wake cycle and all its related processes, which include mood regulation.[28] Our retinas take in information from sunlight and use it to send messages to our brain, which is why it's so essential our eyes get that message from natural daylight.

Unfortunately, the last hundred years or so has seen us humans exist indoors more and more, and rely on artificial light, which simply doesn't have the same effects – and which can have a detrimental effect on our mood. Not only that, but we are taught to fear the sun, with constant doom-and-gloom news about the risks of skin cancer and the advice to slather ourselves in SPF all year round. Anyone who dares contradict this comes in for all sorts of criticism – Professor Tim Spector recently made the point that too much sun protection can 'block our natural defences' and 'wearing SPF 50 for 365 days a year is likely excessive and likely to leave [people] vitamin D deficient'.[29] This didn't go down well *at all*. Personally, I just don't think vitamin D supplements in isolation are enough, but if you are relying on them, be sure your vitamin D is D3, vitamin MK-7, along with magnesium L-Threonate and be sure to take it in the morning as it is a stimulant. You don't want it keeping you up all night.

The longevity benefits of sunlight

I'm not claiming there isn't a skin cancer risk from excessive sun damage – especially if you have a family history of melanoma, or are extremely pale and freckly. But honestly, I believe we are told so much BS about the sun, as if it's a 'new' thing instead of something we have evolved to co-exist with! I'm always out in the sun and I certainly don't put SPF all over me, and my data from the Lanserhof clinic showed me that my skin is really healthy. Of course, maybe I'm lucky (however, I very much doubt that it's luck and more so strategy) and my skin has a tolerance to sunlight, but as Dr Vincent Esposito has pointed out, 'the sun gives life to every being on this planet . . . lack of sunlight is human's #1 nutrient deficiency'.[30] It might be worth noting that the majority of deadly skin cancers are *not* caused by sun exposure and are in random places like the soles of the feet and other areas that don't tend to be exposed.

There is still so much to learn about skin cancers, but dermatologists are increasingly conflicted about the role of the sun in causing them. Of course, getting sunburnt is going to cause inflammation, which is never good, so I would recommend shade and light cotton clothes in peak sunlight hours. I would also recommend mineral-based sunscreens (bizarrely called inorganic) over the chemically laden 'organic' sunscreens that contain known carcinogens. Otherwise, ensuring consistent sun exposure – outside of those peak hours, all year round – is going to help keep your vitamin D up and your stress down. The way this works is that UV light from the sun interacts with cholesterol under the skin to produce Vitamin D. Another interesting fact I didn't know about cholesterol!

Interestingly, studies are now under way looking at how nicotinamide (vitamin B3) is highly effective at reducing UV-induced immune suppression, aka reduction in skin cancer. Vitamin B3 can be found in grape seeds,[31] which makes you wonder if genetically modified seedless grapes have actually impacted our skin health, particularly as they are native to the Mediterranean where sun exposure is high. I know I'm going to be opting for seeded grapes from now on.

Sunlight brings us so many health and longevity benefits – it lowers our blood pressure, prevents some cancers, improves metabolic response and balances our hormones.[32] It helps us improve our mood and deal with stress by releasing serotonin, and by stimulating vitamin D, which also has incredible effects on our mental health – there is an 8–14 per cent higher risk of depression in people with vitamin D deficiency.[33]

Other benefits of vitamin D include improved:
- immunity
- autophagy
- cognition and mood
- bone health
- eye health
- sleep patterns

We all know that we naturally feel better on sunny days, don't we? Even on a cloudy day our bodies and brains still pick up the signals from the sun. So – I'll keep saying it for ever – get outside every morning and let daylight do its mood-boosting, de-stressing magic. Even on a gloomy day there is light information to be absorbed, and a recent study showed that people who spend more time outside, regardless of the weather, have a lower BMI. Fun fact, vitamin D is actually a hormone.

What about red-light therapy?

Red-light therapy has become more accessible over the years and is a great way to supplement natural daylight – which of course is extra-important for us living in northerly climes, where abundant sunlight can be hard to come by during the winter months! Red-light therapy uses what's called *light-emitting diodes* (LEDs) to transmit infrared/red light into our body's cells.[34] It works because it activates our cell's mitochondria (engine room) and therefore stimulates anti-inflammatory functions like muscle recovery and healing, pain relief and production of collagen.[35]

On the stress-busting front, red and infrared light is thought to help improve mood as it mimics those key wavelengths of sunlight that do such a brilliant job. Although more peer-reviewed research needs to be done, one small study showed that infrared light applied to the forehead had a positive effect on people suffering from depression, with no side effects.[36]

You can rent a red light to go on your desk at work or have at home. You can buy portable infrared saunas off Amazon – I use mine all the time (sitting in there watching telly, *naturally*) although they are still a bit of an investment piece (approximately £200, but as I use it

---

most days that is less than £1 a go). Infrared LED masks are also now incredibly popular for their skin-improving qualities (and you'll benefit from enhanced mood, too). If you can't stretch to buying either, lots of gyms offer infra-red saunas you can use, or you can book a session at a local spa.

2. Temperature

It's fabulous to lean into activities that put your body under good amounts of stress, such as hot and cold exposure. These days, everyone knows about the mental health benefits of things like cold-water swimming (so much so that wearing Dryrobes has become a bit of a middle-aged cliché!), but the facts are the facts: putting our bodies under heat or cold stressors is highly beneficial, reducing inflammation and sparking dopamine and serotonin release.[37]

We can access this super-easily, from blasting ourselves in a cold shower or sitting in a sauna (see above) and pushing ourselves to stay in for a little longer than is comfortable. Developing a tolerance for stress in this way – by 'microdosing' the stress – can be good for us, because like with exercise, our bodies learn how to buffer it and recover faster, which is the key for managing healthy cortisol levels.[38]

I like to get a sweat on in the evening and sit in my infra-red sauna, because it brings me right down into a cosy, calm state. Obviously, we sweat in saunas, and that has an indirectly positive effect on our livers, too. When we sweat out more toxins via our skin, we leave our livers free to spend more time on other metabolic functions.[39] I find it fascinating that all these bodily functions, like crying and sweating, are nature's ways of detoxing ourselves from stress ... Remember a clear liver means better hormone health: we detox toxic oestrogen via the liver. I love my daft-looking sauna pod and watch some TV while enjoying it every night. It feels like a glass of wine replacement!

3. Connection

We humans are social beings, and connecting with others is vital for balancing our mood. Seeing our friends and having a rant, catching up with our partner, going to the supermarket and chatting with the cashier – whatever it is, we need to connect with others. People with more connections to others not only are happier, with higher self-esteem, but are less likely to suffer with anxiety and depression, and live longer.[40] Social isolation is now understood to be a massive factor in early death.[41]

As well as getting out there into the world, we can also de-stress ourselves by thinking about the big picture: connecting ourselves to the universe. Now, I am the last person to go fully woo-woo, but there really is something in the ability to let go and understand that not everything is within your control. It honestly presses a magic de-stress button!

Put it like this: imagine the traffic is crap, you're stuck in the car and you're going to be late. Our default response might be to feel super-stressed out – catastrophising about the delay, feeling anxious and panicky, and therefore spiking our stress hormones. We all know what that feels like, don't we?

What I've tried to do recently when things like this happen is to hand it over. Hand over the responsibility of the stress and think about the situation differently. Reframe it. So instead of getting super-frustrated that I'm stuck in traffic, I'll think, *OK, this is what the universe wants for me in this situation. Maybe I'm in this traffic now so I won't get into a car crash later down the road.* Typical me, extreme and dramatic. Could just be I don't get flashed on a speed camera.

By leaning into it, understanding that there are things happening that are beyond my control, it just makes me feel like my shoulders have dropped down by about a foot! I relax down into the situation and go *Ahhhh.* Things will always go wrong (and especially for me in the mornings, when I try and pack far too much in), so I find it's helpful to mentally let go and trust in the situation. If something is beyond your control, it's beyond your control! We may as well let go, sit back and go, *OK, fine.* For now, it's teaching me to let go.

The biggest stress-relieving life lesson

On a similar note, another brilliant 'let it go' lesson I've learned is realising that nobody gives a shit what you're doing. A lot of this may be down to getting older (and a tiny bit wiser), but whatever age we are, it is so freeing to realise that nobody out there in the real world is out there to judge *you*, because they're all locked into their own heads. We don't have to be 'perfect', to look a certain way with a face full of make-up. We don't have to worry about looking like a newbie in the gym, because nobody is looking at us. They're there for themselves; you are not that important. It's like going to your first party sober and freaking out about what everyone's reaction is going to be. You realise pretty quickly that nobody notices after their first glass of wine. Everybody is in their *own tunnel and ARE NOT going to remember what you're saying anyway. Once the drunk monologue has been activated, prepare to be bored, in over-familiar clutches, endless repetition and showers of spittle.*

Knowing this is such a great relief. Have a think about it: the last time you went out, what was everyone else wearing? You will have no fucking idea at all, because you wouldn't have noticed; you were probably too busy thinking about what *you* were doing, wearing or saying. And that's the same for everyone else. Realising that we are not that important to the general populace is so freeing. So, stop worrying about not having the perfect make-up or handbag or whatever, because nobody else gives a shit, in the nicest possible way. For me, this little gem of knowledge is brilliant for stress relief. Also backdoor at parties, say bye to the host and swerve the rest. You will save hours on godawful small talk and bullshit promises to meet up soon. We need our sleep!

Why running is my de-stressing lifeline

If you follow me on Instagram, you'll already know just how important running is to me, and have seen enough of my sweaty posts that you're probably like, *Yeah, I get it, you love running* by now! But I want to mention it again here, not as a fitness protocol but as a stress-relieving personal mental health *necessity*. I'm not exaggerating when I say it bolsters my self-esteem in such a profound way that I could not do without it.

When I started running, it was a big struggle – not least because I had to stop all the time to go for a frigging wee! (I was living in London at the time and running around Hyde Park – I promise I can still recall where every single public loo was because I had to go in them all the time, yep, even the most dubious ones . . .) But within such a short space of time, I was running longer and longer distances, feeling better physically and mentally, and yep, even managing to run past the loos without having to use them! I did the Manchester Marathon with one loo stop in five hours of running and chatting (yeah . . . I even talk there).

Whatever your level of fitness, a small amount of effort with running leads to monumental gains. Running gives me a sense of freedom and confidence that improves every single one of my day-to-day activities and interactions. I know I can cope better with things after a run that would otherwise have pissed me off big-time. Running is my lifeline, and so if you haven't tried it yet, I urge you to do so.

4. Downtime

How we choose to spend our downtime is a deeply personal choice. Like I mentioned earlier, what is relaxing to one person is a stressful nightmare to another! Many of you will already know that I love to binge-watch telly as my go-to relaxation. Loads of us do – it's not exactly an unusual, niche hobby, is it? – but I strongly feel *what* I watch is so important in order to properly balance my stress levels.

My criteria: it needs to be something with no trauma, no murder and no sodding real-life-crime plot lines that will resonate in my already frazzled brain. I know how my mind works. If I've had a stressful day, I will naturally be in a dark place; and if I'm confronted with the worst of humanity, even if it's fictional, I'll go even further down that bleak hole and traumatise myself. I'm not immune to the news, or the worst parts of social media, so I need to protect myself psychologically, stay resilient and not watch things that make me feel despondent about life. We *all* do.

The de-stressing distraction of bullshit TV

This is why I think bullshit TV – by which I mean dump-your-brain-at-the-door reality shows – has a place. It doesn't matter how highbrow your tastes usually are, or your level of education – in this era of whatever-you-want streaming, we all need to look at the content we expose ourselves to. If we're overworked, or in a sensitive place, watching something that is mentally and emotionally taxing won't do us any favours. Sometimes you just need to gawp at a load of strangers on telly and think, *Ooh, that dress looks awful on her* or *That person's skin looks fantastic!* – something as stupid and bland as that can just help you come out of the funk.

For me, this is one of the most effective ways to truly switch off. To rest and reset, to calm the hell down before I go to sleep. Our brains are overloaded and our cortisol is being constantly spiked by modern life, so we need these places where we can be completely passive, be taken out of our daily stresses and be entertained *without* effort. The stakes are low, there is no controversy, nothing for us to get wound up about, which is *perfect*. The brain-dead stuff is what we need to reset our brains, and anyone who passes judgement clearly doesn't have enough plates to spin!

So, whatever it is you like to do in your downtime – whether it's telly watching, reading, listening to podcasts, walking, whatever – give yourself permission to truly switch off when you engage with it. If something winds you up, just flipping avoid it! Lean into the things that resonate with *you*, that you find relaxing. Do not feel shame about it. I've found my perfect downtime happy place and it's watching bullshit TV (my favourite is *Married at First Sight*; for another friend, it's *The Pioneer Woman* on the Food Network). So whatever works for you is the right choice. My husband ends up into it too, so it's a bit of quality time together.

My top five calm-the-f----down takeaways

So much of what we've covered so far in this book will really help in reducing your stress response – eating anti-inflammatory foods (good fats, good protein, less starchy carbs), muscle-building and staying mobile; all of these are absolutely guaranteed to help improve your mental resilience. Hoo-bloody-ray. And what we've zoomed in on with this final chapter is how important it is to be tuned into our stress levels because they are an essential principle for better healthspan and longevity.

When lots of mini stressors build up over our days, weeks, months and years, we end up with what Mo Gawdat, author of *Unstressable*, calls 'excessive wear and tear on our biological systems'. Other experts like Dr Lawson Wulsin, the author of *Toxic Stress*, have said that 'stress deserves to be a top public health priority', because, simply put, it can kill us.[42] Understanding this is the first step in making sure we put the spotlight on stress. It's not woo-woo nonsense, it's vital to our health and as important as nutrition and exercise. There are loads of tips in this chapter and, like I said, I think it's important to make them personal and meaningful for you. But I believe that everyone can adapt and make use of the top five tips below:

1. **Cut down on booze**. It's a fake friend. It spikes our cortisol when we don't need it and ruins sleep.
2. **Support your natural cortisol boost**. Tackle your stressful tasks in the morning, and supplement with Relora & L-theanine if you need it.
3. **Use the double inhalation breathing technique** to buffer stress in five seconds.
4. **Get outside**: sunlight, running and connection are the ultimate free de-stressors.
5. **Make your evening truly relaxing** by considering the content you're exposed to and keeping lights low. Bring out the non-toxic candles and blue-light blocking glasses.

FUTUREPROOF LIVING: PUTTING IT INTO ACTION

If you've read everything so far up until this point, thank you. Welcome to the last part and well bloody done! I massively appreciate you spending the time reading through each chapter. However, if you've skipped to this part first because you just want to know what to buy and what to do, welcome too! (Like you, I often do this because I'm impatient and sometimes I cannot be arsed with doing things the long way round.)

Whichever route you've taken to get here, this is the section where I'll show you the steps to apply all the Futureproof Principles to your life, in the most actionable, achievable way possible. We've covered off so many tips and takeaways that there's no way I'd expect you to be able to apply them all at once

— that would be insane and a one-way ticket to a complete and utter breakdown. We can all make positive changes to our lives, but I understand how overwhelming it can feel at the start. I live in the real world and I *get it* – of course, you'll have all your usual responsibilities of work, family, friends, hobbies, errands, food shopping, getting the cat de-fleaed. Whatever you normally need to get done isn't going to disappear, just so you can start on a new healthy action plan, is it? Nope.

So, this section has been designed to work around regular life – whatever that looks like for you. We're going to spend some time getting **Futureproof Ready** with a week of planning activities. We're going to look at a **Futureproof Supplements** list, including those that are readily available and those that you need to keep your eye on for the future! And then we're going to look at some different **Futureproof Daily Schedules** depending on the day you're having.

I've done this because none of us lives through *exactly* the same day repeated over and over again (despite how things can feel sometimes, we don't live in *Groundhog Day*!). Some days we have the time and space and mental energy to really prioritise our health. Other days we are frantically busy with work or kids or other commitments. Some days we haven't slept properly or are just in a terrible mood. Some days we're away from home and trying to work with a completely different set of temptations and priorities. That's just life and we need to work around it, so we're going to plan for (most) eventualities.

A quick note about the key: I've tagged each piece of advice, supplement or protocol with a **FP1, FP2, FP3, FP4** or **FP5**. These correlate to the chapters we've covered and support the main principles within those chapters:

FP1 – fights inflammation
FP2 – supports muscle-building
FP3 – prioritises protein
FP4 – maximises moving
FP5 – balances stress

So, for example, something with the code FP1 will carry a piece of advice that supports reducing inflammation. Got it? *Fab.*

Futureproof Living isn't about being super-disciplined every second, and then feeling like a failure when you don't live up to these high expectations. We're not having any of that! Whatever you can do, I applaud. These plans are designed to be achievable for all of us, whatever's going on in our lives. Remember, it's about progress, not perfection, *always.* (This phrase was taught to me by someone much wiser than me – so keep it in mind, always!)

(1) GET FUTUREPROOF READY: A WEEK TO PLAN

I've included this section as planning is absolutely essential! There are a lot of moving parts when it comes to making positive changes in your life; it's not just a plug-in-and-go situation, is it? So, here are some ideas for how to go about getting your home, work and life Futureproof Ready in one week.

I've given each weekday a shortish job to do so that you can fit it around your daily commitments and put the more time-consuming stuff in on the weekend days, assuming that you'll have more time free then. However, if this doesn't work for you, feel free to mix it up. This is just a framework, so please do season to your own personal taste . . .

Monday

One hour: Online shop prep

- Open up your last online grocery shop or saved shopping list. Look through your list for any UPFs and delete them off your list – if they're not there, you won't buy them!
  - FYI, the brilliant Dr Cate Shanahan has categorised what constitutes a UPF: anything that contains vegetable oil, refined grains, refined sugar and crap processed proteins like milk protein, whey protein, pea protein, brown rice protein, textured vegetable protein
  - Vegetable/seed oils include: rapeseed, sunflower, corn etc., soy
  - Sweeteners include: sucralose, aspartame, acesulfame potassium
  - Thickeners include: carrageenan, guar, xantham gums
  - Stabilisers include: maltodextrin, lecithin, E numbers *(FP1)*
- Swap the below for an alternative:
  - Breaded fish/chicken for salmon or chicken fillet (with the skin on!) and an added herb crust
  - Fruit juices/smoothies for whole fruit
  - Potatoes for aubergine/cauliflower/peppers/squash/celeriac
  - Sweetened plant milk for whole milk, cream, raw milk or Jersey cows A2 milk
  - Sweetened fruit yogurt for plain full-fat Greek yogurt
  - Diet or full-fat fizzy drinks for sparkling water and kombucha (ideally made by independent producers

rather than the big fizzy-drink manufacturers)
- o Milk chocolate biscuits for bars of dark chocolate (70 per cent+ cocoa) or WillPowders protein powder
- o Crisps for olive-oil-baked crackers
- o Sliced processed bread for sourdough loaf *(FP1, FP2, FP3)*
- Make sure you include:
- o Saturated fats aka stable fats for cooking: olive oil, avocado oil, ghee or butter
- o Full-fat dairy: yogurt, cheese, milk, cottage cheese
- o Meat and fish: fatty cuts of beef, chicken, salmon, cod (all skin on)
- o Non-meat items: eggs, avocados, chickpeas, tempeh, lentils (if you're using dried beans, leave soaking for many hours before cooking to reduce lectins)
- o Snack superheroes: Peanut butter, nuts, berries *(FP1, FP2, FP3)*
- Meal plan three dinners that prioritise protein and add the ingredients onto your list *(FP2, FP3).*

Tuesday

Thirty minutes: Office sort-out

Whether you're WFH or in an office . . .

- Move your office bin far enough away that you need to walk to it.
- Reschedule any regular high-pressure meetings to the mornings.
- Look into buying a portable full-spectrum infrared panel light for your desk to boost dopamine and improve your mood.

- Put in at least a thirty-minute 'busy' period each day on your digital work calendar for you to eat your lunch and get outdoors *(FP4, FP5)*.
- Search online for a widget that uses the Pomodoro Technique (twenty-five minutes working, five-minute break) and install it on your work computer *(FP4, FP5)*.

If you work in an office . . .

- Email HR or your line manager and ask for a workstation assessment *(FP4)*.
- Ask them about standing desks, screen height and footrests *(FP4)*.

Wednesday

One hour: Workout groundwork

- Research local gyms online and shortlist up to three that you could easily get to.
- Message local friends who go to the gym. Ask them:
  - How much they cost
  - What facilities they have
  - What's the vibe?
  - When do they go and how do they fit it in?
  - What offers they have for new members *(FP2, FP4)*
- Call or email at least one gym (preferably two so you can compare) and book in a visit or trial session *(FP1, FP2)*.
- Check through your kit and make sure you have:
  - Gym wear that fits and feels comfy (it doesn't need to be fancy!)

o Trainers that fit well and support your feet
o Earphones/earbuds and a belt/arm strap to hold your phone in place *(FP2)*

If you really can't go to the gym:

- Grab a notepad and stretch out . . .
- Take your baseline info: log your stats for weight-free muscle-builders:
  o Push-ups done in one minute
  o Wall squat maximum time
  o Plank maximum time
- Set a reminder on your phone for a weekly check-in to update these figures and to share with a couple of other mates.
- Search online for affordable skipping ropes, dumbbells and kettlebell weights. Look on eBay, Gumtree and Vinted for second-hand, or ask around your mates for cast-offs! *(FP2, FP5).*

Thursday
Thirty minutes: Bedroom blitz

- Open up your windows and air the space.
- Got any house plants? Move at least one into your bedroom.
- Any air fresheners? Chuck them out. Scented candles containing paraffin wax, soy, synthetic fragrances, dyes? Do the same.
- Check: are your sheets made of cotton? If not, order

some new ones (or add to a birthday wish list! Organic if you can . . .)

- Dig out that old alarm clock and set it ten minutes earlier than your usual alarm.
- Look into a grounding mat for the bed. I've had one for ages and I wrote about it in my first book.
- If you watch telly in bed, check the angle and move the TV to make sure you're not misaligned or straining your body *(FP1, FP4, FP5)*.

Friday

Thirty minutes: Power playlists

- Create three music playlists on your phone for different circumstances:
  - On the way rev-up – pre-workout tunes that make you feel happy and positive
  - Full-on workout – hi-energy, hi-BPM music, whether house, rock, pop or rap
  - Chilled cardio – mid-tempo tracks for a relaxing run *(FP2, FP4, FP5)*
- Share it with friends on social media and ask for any track recommendations *(FP2, FP5)*.

Saturday

One hour plus: Kitchen clear-out

- *Dump the veg oil:* look at the ingredients list on all the products in your fridge, freezer and cupboards and see if they contain veg oils.

- Chuck them out if you are able to, but if not, make a note of the offenders and stick it on your fridge to ensure you don't buy them again! (NB Don't pour veg oil down the drain as it creates fatbergs – *heave*.) *(FP1, FP3, FP5)*.
- *Clean up your cleaners* – look at your cleaning products and consider getting rid of any which include pesticides: commonly ending with '–onium chloride' e.g. benzalkonium chloride *(FP1, FP3)*.
- Look up eco-friendly alternatives and add to your shop, or buy some distilled white vinegar (only about a tenner from Amazon for a huge 5l bottle) and use that instead. Much cheaper and better for you *(FP1, FP3)*.
- *Get ahead of your cravings* – prep some healthy sweet treats to keep in the freezer:
  o No-churn ice cream: mix vanilla or chocolate protein powder with Greek yogurt and freeze
  o If you have an ice-cream maker: full-fat milk, double cream, vanilla or chocolate protein powder, churn! Add activated nuts and a pinch of salt for extra satisfaction.

Sunday

One hour plus: Bathroom balance

- *Detoxify your skin:* Chuck out aluminium-based deodorants and perfumes and replace with (or order) a new eco non-chemical one (I like Wild). It is definitely trial and error as some leave a deodorant mark! *(FP1, FP3)*

225

- *Clean up your cleaners* – look at your bathroom cleaning products the same way you did in the kitchen. Big culprits commonly containing pesticides and/or heavy metals like aluminium are nail-polish remover and toilet cleaner *(FP1, FP3)*.
- Check your towels are 100 per cent cotton and if they're not, and you can afford to, replace them! TK Maxx is ace for this!
- *Improve mobility:* Put a small footstool or toddler step next to your toilet *(FP4)*.

End-of-the-week treat:

Book yourself either an infrared/regular sauna *(FP1, FP5)*, infrared facial *(FP1, FP5)*, or an NRT session *(FP4)* and congratulate yourself on a week well done.

(2)
FUTUREPROOF SUPPLEMENTS LIST

Readily available supplements (UK)

Speak to a doctor if you're on any pharmaceutical medicine that might have an interaction with any of these supplements. (For example, berberine thins the blood which may interact with blood-thinning medications like aspirin.)

Berberine – bioactive compound lowers blood-sugar levels, regulates metabolism, reduces heart disease and can help alleviate depression[1] *(FP1, FP5)*

Black cumin-seed oil – has anti-inflammatory and skin-boosting properties, and may help maintain healthy weight[2] *(FP1, FP2, FP3)*

Collagen powder – amino-acid peptides boost collagen production, supporting immune system, muscle synthesis and skin health *(FP1, FP2, FP3)*

Creatine – amino-acid compound, great for powering muscles and improved brain function *(FP2, FP3)*

Curcumin (turmeric) – alleviates oxidative stress and reduces inflammation, especially in muscles post-exercise[3] *(FP1, FP2)*

Glycine – amino acid which counters oxidative stress, supports skin health, protects heart, helps build muscle *(FP1, FP2, FP3, FP5)*

Licorice root – has anti-inflammatory properties and can help with skin conditions *(FP1, FP3)*

L-theanine – amino acid which helps regulate mood, decrease stress and promote good sleep *(FP5) works in fifteen minutes*

Magnesium – brilliant all-rounder mineral, great for muscle–protein synthesis, reducing stress and inflammation, great taken in the morning. There are lots of different types of magnesium that support different functions, so I have included a cheat sheet below *(FP1, FP2, FP3, FP5)*

NAC+ – anti-inflammatory amino acids, help regulate blood glucose and muscle–protein synthesis *(FP1, FP2, FP3)*

Relora – bark extract that helps maintain healthy cortisol levels *(FP5) works in four weeks*

Resveratrol – bioactive compound with anti-oxidant and anti-inflammatory effects, protective against many chronic diseases[4] *(FP1)*

Silica – essential trace element which makes collagen more bioavailable, supporting skin/hair health *(FP3)*

Tart cherry extract – anti-inflammatory and reduces muscle soreness *(FP1, FP2)*

Vitamin C – supports collagen production, opt for natural acerola extract *(FP3)*

Vitamin D – great for reducing musculoskeletal pain as well as improving bone health, mood and disease risk. Best taken in the morning *(FP2, FP5)*.

Magnesium Cheat Sheet

Glycinate = Sleep and relaxation

Malate = Muscle and energy

Turate = Heart and blood pressure

Theronate = Cognition and memory

Orotate = Heart and muscle

Sulfate = Muscle soreness (Applied topically. Do not consume.)

Citrate = Constipation (Use in the bath. Do not consume.)

Chloride = Digestion and dehydration

Stuff that's a little bit out there / on the horizon . . .

Peptides

IVs e.g. High dose vitamin C

EB02

Hyperbaric oxygen therapy

CRISPR (this is a form of gene editing which is currently hugely controversial but has been shown to be effective against certain diseases)

(3)
FUTUREPROOF
DAILY
SCHEDULES

Five different ways to adapt the Futureproof protocols in a twenty-four-hour period, depending which sort of day you're having!

The *Perfect* Day

For those lovely times when you can plan your day to support Futureproof Living – rather than the other way around . . .

First thing:

Get outside and on to a grounding mat or towel (which contain copper ions, helping to conduct the earth's magnetic field). Grounding helps with regulating your sleep cycle, reducing inflammation, pain and stress.[5] If you don't have one, just walk around barefoot outside for a little while. Drink a glass of electrolytes (water with added lemon juice and sea salt) while you soak in any sunshine for twenty minutes. Even in overcast weather your brain will get the benefits. *(FP1, FP4, FP5)*

Breakfast:

When everything's going well is a great time to promote autophagy and reduce inflammation with intermittent fasting. Give your body a rest, so drink an MCT coffee with added collagen powder, and feed your brain with a nootropic supplement like L-theanine, which will give you a calm, focused energy. *You'll be pushing your body to become fat adapted. (FP1, FP3, FP5)*

Morning:

Get moving and muscle-building! This is the perfect time to go for a run, a ruck (weighted backpack walk) or for a session at the gym – exercising promotes a healthy release of cortisol, which is great in the morning when it naturally peaks, and of course helps reduce inflammation and improve muscle synthesis, as well as blitzing stress levels. Get those uplifting tunes going, sunglasses off and get into the zone. *(FP1, FP2, FP4, FP5)*

If you're really starving after your workout, have a decent protein shake made with raw milk, or a bowl of Greek yogurt with some activated nuts and berries to reduce the delayed-onset muscle soreness. *(FP3)*

Lunchtime:

Have some fermented food first off to reduce inflammation and promote gut biodiversity – either with a kombucha, spoonful of kimchi or kefir yogurt. You can try trimethylglycine to reduce any histamine response to fermented foods or bone broth. Your gut will eventually heal and the histamine response should reduce. *(FP1)*

Prioritise protein for your first meal of the day – eggs are a brilliant option which are incredibly quick to cook. Great options could include scrambled egg with smoked salmon, poached eggs with avocado, three-egg omelette with cheese, or a protein pancake: three eggs, two scoops of bone-broth protein and whipped cream and blueberries fried in ghee or butter. Because this is the perfect day, we're going to avoid bread for now . . . *(FP3)*

Afternoon:

Take a few minutes to practise your mobilisations: the sit-and-get-up test and squatting, and balancing on one leg. *(FP4)*

Avoid the temptation to pick at sweet things and instead stave off any cravings with Greek yogurt, some nuts, bone broth with butter, MCT oil and salt or protein drink. *(FP3, FP5)*

Dinner:

On this perfect day, you've got the time to make a lovely home-cooked meal that's protein-first, right? (Indulge me – this is an ideal world . . .) If you want carbs, these are best enjoyed now, too, as they promote the sleep hormone melatonin. Ride the carb coma to bed (and maybe add in a shot of apple cider vinegar mixed with water as a precursor to dinner if you're sensitive to a glucose spike). Recipe ideas could include:

- Roast dinner with veg and bone-broth gravy
- Steak with air-fryer sweet potato chips
- Salmon with puy lentils and salad
- Skin-on chicken with sourdough and salad *(FP3, FP5)*

Sit on the floor while watching TV *(FP4)* or, even better, meet up with a friend for a good old rant and decompression session. *(FP5)*

Before bed:

Take some magnesium glycinate, L-Theanine, chamomile tea with extra collagen, and/or tart cherry extract to help with inflammation, recovery and muscle synthesis. *(FP1, FP2)*

Spend some time looking after yourself. Depending on what's available to you, do at least one of the following:

- Fascia roll
- Infrared sauna/LED face mask
- Epsom salt bath followed by cold-water blast
- Wim Hof breathing: breathe in and hold your breath for as long as you can, then breathe out. Repeat for thirty breath cycles. *(FP1, FP4, FP5)*
- Listen to a podcast in the bath
- Journal

The *Away from Home* Day

Whether on holiday, travelling for work or visiting friends, being out of your comfort zone can be tricky. Here's how to Futureproof it anyway:

NB – you'll need to do a bit of forward planning here and bring some Futureproof supplies on your travels. I take sachets of MCT powder/oil, collagen powder, a brain-boosting nootropic blend containing L-theanine, and my gym kit plus headphones with me whenever I travel.

First thing:

You might wake up feeling bloated if you've overdone it on food and drink the night before (more likely if you're on holiday). Give yourself a healthy dose of L-theanine with your morning coffee or tea to avoid those jitters, and add in some collagen or keto powder if you have it to hand.

No whizzer to make your usual MCT coffee? One nice little hack I found was that if you mix all your powders or oils together in an empty cup, then stick it under the coffee machine, that works pretty well in making that creamy coffee. (Or you can just stir like crazy with a teaspoon – whatever works.) *(FP1, FP4, FP5)*

Get outside into the sunshine and resist sticking those sunglasses on – you want to keep your body's cells in their regular sleep–wake cycle and sunlight helps with this. *(FP1, FP5)*

Breakfast:

Dealing with a breakfast buffet and the multiple temptations thereof? Yep, it can be hard when you're faced with wall-to-wall bread, pastries and chocolate cereal, especially if you've gone all-inclusive and want to get your money's worth!

If you've had your MCT coffee already, your cravings should be happily dampened down, but if this isn't the case, the egg station is your friend. Before you get waylaid by the pancakes and dive into the carbs (which will just leave you sluggish for the rest of the day), get yourself an omelette, or some boiled/poached eggs, made fresh if that's available. (However, I'd swerve those catering troughs full of dry, spongey scrambled eggs . . . that's never a good way to start the day.) Bacon and avocado are also great options for protein-fuelled breakfasts. Ask them to cook in butter too! *(FP3)*

Morning:

If you're in sunny climes, get out in the fresh air to boost your vitamin D production. Lie on the grass or sand for fifteen minutes to ground. *(FP1, FP5)*

If there's a gym, get in there for a quick twenty-minute session to raise your dopamine to get you ramped up with enthusiasm for the rest of the day, and give you more energy. If you're working, or with friends and there isn't a gym nearby, do a fast walk between meetings or appointments. *(FP2, FP4)*

Lunchtime:

If you had a decent breakfast buffet earlier, try to give your body a break and promote autophagy. If not (or you're just starving regardless!), prioritise protein, in whatever form you can get it. Chicken, lamb, beef, avocado, eggs, tofu and cheese are all friends. *(FP1, FP2)*

Afternoon:

Make sure you stay hydrated with electrolyte drinks, kombucha or just good old water and salt and get outside – whatever you're doing – to enjoy the rest of the day's sun. If you want to, use a mineral SPF which protects your skin – while letting the sun do its mood-boosting magic – and is free from inflammation-spiking chemicals like parabens, silicones and allergens. I like New Layer, or Shade brands. *(FP1, FP4, FP5)*

Dinner:

Freshly cooked meats and fish on the grill are absolutely brilliant when you're on holiday – and good for you. Have those with a salad or veg on the side and you're sorted. *(FP3)*

If you give in to the breadbasket at your evening meal, or indulge in heavier foods than usual, don't worry. (We all do it, and it's impossible to always avoid!) This is the perfect time to do it because carbs promote serotonin release, which gives you that lovely cosy feeling and promotes the sleep hormone melatonin, and you can ride that carb coma all the way to bed . . .

Before bed:

If you've been drinking, make sure you take a liver-supporting supplement before you go to bed. My company WillPowders produce a specific supplement for this exact occasion which includes ingredients like NAC, Milk Thistle and NADH, which could also be supplemented with individually.

The *Super Busy With Work* Day

Completely run ragged with work deadlines, meetings and tasks? No time to think, let alone do a proper workout and prep a proper meal? No problem.

First thing:

Don't leap straight out of bed, even if you have a million and one things to do. Take sixty seconds while you're still in bed to do some quick breathwork. Once you get up, do some gentle mobilisations in your bedroom (squats, sitting down cross-legged and getting up, stretching out while lying down) to gently activate your body. *(FP2, FP4, FP5)*

Breakfast:

Being super-pressed for time is actually a great excuse for a fast – because it saves you the time of prepping and eating anyway! Fuel your mental and physical energy instead with a quick and easy electrolyte drink – a glass of still water with a squeeze of lemon juice and a pinch of sea salt. The potassium and sodium spark your body's electrical conductors into action, getting you going for a busy day. *(FP1, FP5)*

Have a morning coffee too (with MCT oil/powder) to fuel your brain with good fats, and add some L-theanine supplements so you get a cool calm energy to see you through your busy work schedule. You should feel the positive effects within fifteen to twenty minutes as it lowers your stress and improves cognition . . . All together now, *Ahhhh. (FP1, FP3, FP5)*

Morning:

You're flat out, yep, I hear you. But take a five-minute break from the screen and do some 'deskercises' – the gunslinger (arm stretch with your fingers laced together in a gun pose), neck tilt and chest opener. Hold each one for ten seconds, breathe steadily and repeat. *(FP4)*

Have an MCT coffee or kombucha mid-morning. *(FP1, FP3)*

Lunchtime:

Force yourself to take a ten-minute break and stretch your legs – even if it's just down the corridor in your office. If you can, get outside and walk to the shops to get your lunch. There are some great options (even as part of supermarket meal deals) these days that support a protein-first, carb-light and UPF-free eating. Easy Futureproof grab-and-go supermarket lunch wins could include:

- Pot of two boiled eggs
- Hummus pot with carrot sticks (make sure the hummus is free of vegetable oil)
- Pack of baby cucumbers/peppers
- Packets of plain mixed nuts
- Cans of magnesium water/kombucha/CBD drink
- Salad bowl with chicken/eggs/olives/cheese
- Poké bowl with salmon
- Packet of ready-cooked chicken breast/salt beef/salmon
- Tubs of berries
- Greek yogurt pot
- Biltong *(FP1, FP2, FP3)*

Afternoon:

Repeat the at-desk mobilisations from this morning and get up to make yourself a hot drink – stand on one leg while the kettle boils. *(FP4)*

If you're super-stressed from back-to-back Zooms or too many deadlines, practise the physiological sigh (two hiccupy breaths in, one long breath out). Do it three times and feel your shoulders drop right down. *(FP5)*

Dinner:

Out for a work social and know you'll be drinking? Prep yourself better:

- Have a protein shake before you go out to slow down alcohol absorption.
- Take a supplement containing milk thistle and NAC which reduce inflammation and support liver function.
- Avoid high-alcohol-content drinks and those with sugary mixers like Coke, tonic and lemonade. Opt for soda water instead.
- Alternate each boozy drink with a glass of water (I know this is easier said than done!) *(FP1, FP3, FP5)*

If you're not headed out, but are just absolutely done in, with no more mental or physical energy to cook properly, here are some super-quick and easy dinners to pick up that require zero effort (although check the ingredients list for inflammation-spiking veg oils):

- Ready-cooked rotisserie chicken with salad
- Freshly made soup pot containing lentils, beans, chicken, meat, etc.
- Microwaveable pouch of lentil/veggie curry or dal
- Burrito bowl containing meat/beans, rice and veg
- Stews with beans/chicken/beef *(FP3, FP5)*

Before bed:

Still got more work you want to get done? Don't do it sitting up in bed on your laptop. Work in another room and set an alarm to make sure you finish up with time to do one of the following:

- Watch an episode of something easy and undemanding on TV
- Get into a warm bath with Epsom salts
- Read a favourite book or listen to an audiobook *(FP1, FP5)*

The *Woke Up in a Shitty Mood* Day

Some days we just feel absolutely flipping awful for no good reason. That's OK, we can Futureproof it.

First thing:

Feeling below par/irritable/teary/just plain furious? Get yourself outside grounding as soon as you can. Whether you have a grounding mat to sit on or not, you can access the incredible effects that have been found to improve health – including regulating your circadian rhythm and reducing stress.[1] Just walk outside with bare feet for a few moments and take a few physiological sighs to bring your cortisol down. *(FP1, FP4, FP5)*

Breakfast:

You want to avoid any hangry moments, so give the cereal and toast (or even porridge) a big swerve – it will just mess with your blood-sugar levels and make you raging with carb-craving hunger an hour later. If you can, fat-fast with an MCT coffee, because it will boost your brain power; but if you really can't do it today, do not worry. Have a decent bowl of Greek yogurt, with berries, nuts and/or stevia. Knock up a scrambled egg with butter and salt, too, if you fancy it. *(FP1, FP3, FP5)*

Morning:

Have an MCT coffee or kombucha mid-morning. *(FP1, FP3)*

If you can, get out for a run or a gym session – I find it absolutely brilliant for clearing my head and leaning into my natural, healthy cortisol boost. *(FP2, FP4, FP5)*

Lunchtime:

Nourish yourself with a lunch packed with good fats for brain health and satiety. Something like avocado and bacon salad with quinoa, roast chicken thighs with rice cooked in bone broth, or a big egg-and-cheese omelette will make you feel satisfied without the afternoon slump. *(FP3)*

Afternoon:

Have to embark on the dreaded school run, and deal with all the dickhead drivers and annoying traffic? *I know.* But do what you can to let it go. Remember this isn't important – hand over the responsibility for this to the universe. Breathe out.

Dinner:

Make life easy on yourself and do something super-quick and comforting. (Or get somebody else to make it for you if there's anyone who can.) Now's the time for carbs as they'll make you feel rested and ready for bed – if you can and you want, why not take some sourdough and cheese to bed? Or make a hearty stew with whatever meat and veg you have to hand. Whatever makes you feel better and takes you into a more relaxed state of mind . . .

Before bed:

Take some time to watch some relaxing mood-boosting and brain-dumping telly that makes you feel all cosy and happy. Don't expose yourself to anything that will aggravate, stress or worry you. Sit on the floor with your legs crossed to improve mobility while you do. (FP4, FP5)

The *Day After The Night Before* **Day**

Whether you were out late indulging yourself or just had a shocking sleep for no good reason (it happens), this is for when you haven't had a proper night's rest.

First thing:

Resist the temptation to sleep in later than you usually do even if you're shattered – your cells work on a twenty-four-hour clock, and messing with our sleep–wake cycles will just make it harder to get a good night's sleep later on. So, drag yourself up at your usual time, but make sure to get an early night this evening.

Get some electrolytes into your system – either with a DIY drink (water, pinch of sea salt and squeeze of lemon) or with electrolyte rehydration sachets. Have a shower with a cold blast of water at the end (to stimulate your vagus nerve) and get straight outside to get that sunlight into your eyes. Yes, you may be desperate to hide away under those sunglasses, but fight the urge . . . *(FP1, FP4, FP5)*

Breakfast:

You'll be craving sugar if you haven't slept well, because poor sleep is a *killer* for this – it promotes our hunger hormone ghrelin and suppresses leptin (our satiety neurotransmitter). Gorging on sweet things will only make you feel worse, though – your blood glucose will mess with your energy levels, and remember, sugar creates glycation in collagen, leaving our skin looking saggy and less bouncy.

Instead nourish yourself with eggs, or Greek yogurt with strawberries or raspberries. Boost your vitamin C with citrus fruit. Have magnesium and L-Theanine to get rid of the beer fear. *(FP1, FP2)*

Morning:

Have another electrolytes drink, or an MCT coffee.

241

If it's a work day, keep your energy levels up by stopping work every hour or so to take a five-minute stretch and mobilisation break. Snack on activated nuts or have a bowl of Greek yogurt.

Lunchtime:

If you've been out on the booze, your skin will be mega-dehydrated, inflamed and desperate for some TLC. Drink a glass of water with some apple-cider vinegar in it for a pre-lunch digestive enzyme. Then treat yourself to some collagen-boosting foods, such as soup made with bone broth, ribeye steak or bacon (with eggs) – all are high in glycine which counteracts a histamine response, too.

Afternoon:

If you can, get to a sauna session to sweat out the overindulgence and support liver detox (you'll feel the benefits even if you're not hung-over) . . .

Snack on some pork scratchings – yep, these old-school snacks are high in glycine, too.

Dinner:

Time for cosy carbs! Have some soup with sourdough bread, or something like lamb chops with some sweet potato. Eat a banana or have a banana protein smoothie afterwards to set yourself up for a restorative sleep – carbs promote serotonin, which triggers production of sleep-inducing melatonin. *(FP3, FP5)*

Before bed:

Get into a warm bath with Epsom salts to relax you. Make sure your room is calm, not too hot and nice and dark so you get a decent night's sleep tonight!

CONCLUSION: THE ONE WORD I WANT TO LEAVE YOU WITH . . .

If there's anything I want to leave you feeling at the end of this book, it's *hope*. Hope because, despite all the depressing crap we read in the news, all the latest health scares and horrible statistics, I passionately believe things can – and will – get better. Yes, of course, like the rest of us, I have days where I feel furious and worried about what's coming down the road – hence my occasional rants on Insta! – but I also feel motivated, encouraged and uplifted by all the incredible innovations, discoveries and alternative approaches that brilliant people are constantly unearthing.

Here are just a few things I've come across that have made me go *wow* recently. A robot which kills weeds with lasers, rather than cancer-causing toxic pesticides (see, not all AI is bad!)[1] A light therapy called PDT which can be used to successfully treat cancers – even those that have previously had very poor treatment outcomes.[2] An incredible caregiver programme which actually reduces cognitive decline in Alzheimer's sufferers.[3]

Every day I read incredible things like this, which make me feel so much more positive about the future. There is more and more coming out every day, and I for one find it completely inspiring. Because learning from the best experts out there has turned my life around. And it's not just about out-there science that's a few years away from impacting our lives. There are brilliant developments everywhere we look – such as the amazing work going on in regenerative farming, which is now hitting our supermarket shelves in the form of sourdough bread! This particular range is made with flour without using herbicides or pesticides. You can buy a loaf for just a couple of quid, and by doing so, you're investing in agriculture that replenishes soil biodiversity and eating proper bread which is brilliant for us (oh, and tastes bloody amazing too). *Fantastic.*

In this book, I wanted to pass along everything I've learned about ageing well and how we can live a long, healthy, vibrant life to the best of our abilities. I wanted to open our minds to new possibilities and new approaches to the science of ageing. I wanted to shift our thinking about getting older, so we're excited about the second half of our lives, rather than dreading it. I wanted to give us actionable insights and real evidence-based advice that we can apply to our everyday lives, even when it's pissing down outside and we're in a crap mood! I hope – yep, that word again – that it helps you Futureproof your life. Try as many of the tips and protocols in this book that you can and let me know how you get on @daviniataylor.

Above all, I wanted to share the knowledge that we can *all* shift our mindsets, make positive changes and live a fabulous life. Because if I can, anyone can.

Davinia xx

RECOMMENDED SUPPLIERS

I'm often asked on Instagram for specific supplier recommendations and, while these are changing all the time, I chose to include a list below similar to the one in my previous books to give you a sense of where I do my own health and biohacking shopping.

I can't mention supplements and suppliers without giving a shoutout to my own business, WillPowders! I started WillPowders in 2021 with the aim of bringing together the best ingredients to produce the most practical and bioavailable nutrition and supplements on the market, and I'm so proud of our products. I remain constantly inquisitive and am always evolving the range, so check out www.willpowders.com for products that have been developed specifically to target the health issues we might be facing.

In addition to my own business there are so many others out there that I believe in, have bought from and find inspirational. Some of my favourite suppliers are listed below and I hope that these resources will help you identify what's right for you and your lifestyle choices.

Online Food Services

planetorganic.co.uk

wholefoodsmarket.co.uk

weareheylo.com

fieldandflower.co.uk

oddbox.co.uk

gazegillorganics.co.uk

abelandcole.co.uk

eversfield-organic.co.uk

thefishsociety.co.uk

riverford.co.uk

fishforthought.co.uk

shop.rickstein.com

ocado.com

Raw Dairy

naturaler.co.uk – for local dairy farms near you

Fermented Food And Drink

lovingfoods.co.uk

myfermentedfoods.com

thesourdoughco.com

superloaf.co.uk

bottlebrushferments.com

labrewery.co.uk

kombuchawarehouse.com

Protein Powders

Bone Broth Protein Powder at willpowders.com

Ancient Nutrition at iherb.com

planetpaleo.co

Protein at gardenoflife.co.uk

Collagen

willpowders.com (grass-fed bovine collagen peptides)

hunterandgatherfoods.com (grass-fed bovine collagen peptides)

ossaorganic.com (grass-fed bovine collagen peptides)

re-coll.co.uk (Beauty collagen)

Vegan Naked Collagyn at ancientandbrave.com

Bone Broth

planetpaleo.co

drgusnutrition.co.uk

Electrolytes

ElectroTide at willpowders.com

E-Lyte at bodybio.co.uk

Nootropics

Pure C8 MCT Oil at willpowders.com

Brain Powder and Calm at willpowders.com

troscriptions.com

dirteaworld.com

Supplements

Full range at willpowders.com

Designs for Health range at supplementhub.co.uk

thorne.com

highernature.com

viridian-nutrition.com

pippacampbellhealth.com

Testing And Equipment

Testing
glycanage.com

omnos.me

thriva.co

lifecodegx.com

medichecks.com

letsgetchecked.co.uk

freestyle.abbott– continuous glucose monitor

hum2n.com

Equipment
redlightrising.com – red lights

functionalself.co.uk – general biohacking store

aquatru.co.uk – reverse osmosis water system

berkey-waterfilters.co.uk – water filters

ouraring.com – health tracker

whoop.com – health tracker

firzone.co.uk – infrared pop-up sauna

infraredsauna.co.uk – infrared sauna for 2+ people

brassmonkey.co.uk - ice baths

discovermonk.com - ice baths

dryrobe.com – changing robe

voited.co.uk – changing robe

ikea.com – chill pad

eightsleep.com – sleep fitness technology

lumen.me

ACKNOWLEDGEMENTS

This book is my way of giving back to my incredible community who give me so much support and energy. You're like family to me and I care about each and every one of you. All I want is for my readers to feel empowered in their own decisions about their health and able to make the right, informed choices. None of us want to end this life feeling defeated and unable to enjoy our later years. It is my hope that the tools and information in this book will help you to avoid just that and, if you're reading this, I hope you'll pass this book to someone you care about. Let's all get optimistic about our health and ready to take action.

Special thanks has to go to my manager and friend Becca Barr. You believed in me before anyone else and I will never forget that. We've achieved so much together, and I feel so lucky to have you in my corner, backing my message all the way.

A big thank you has to go to Becky Howard, who has been invaluable in the process of writing this book. The way you help me get my health philosophy down on the page is literally like magic and I'm so grateful. Gratitude also goes to Jess and the whole team at Orion for helping me bring this longevity message to life and getting this book to the people who need it most. Not to forget the amazing team on the cover shoot. That includes Jessica Hart, Catherine Harbour, Emma Pottinger,

Gemma Sheppard and Cassie Lomas. We had such a laugh, and I think we created something fab!

Behind the scenes I have my amazing WillPowders gang keeping this whole machine running, cheering me along and nurturing this amazing business we are building together. I couldn't do what I do without you all, and I know we're just getting started.

My best mates have to get a shout out. To you girls who try out all my mad tricks and advice – I love you. We're getting healthier together and that is an amazing thing. I want you all with me for the long haul.

Now I come to my gorgeous family, and it makes me genuinely emotional thinking about how much I love and appreciate you. The most special mention to my precious husband Matthew and my adorable sons who give me the courage to keep fighting the good fight, knowing I'll always come home to our safe bubble of chaos. We're living the good life together and I can't wait for everything we have to come.

Matthew, you're my rock, my guiding light and my best mate. Thank you.

And finally, thanks to my mum. Losing you was the toughest thing I've ever been through. I hope you can see me now turning that grief into the energy I needed to become the woman, the mother and the entrepreneur we always knew I could be. I love you and I'll see you on the other side xxx

NOTES

Introduction: How Old Are You Really?

1 https://www.nm.org/healthbeat/medical-advances/science-and-research/What-is-Your-Actual-Age

2 https://www.kingsfund.org.uk/publications/whats-happening-life-expectancy-england

3 https://www.verywellmind.com/alcoholism-as-a-disease-63292

4 https://www.ncbi.nlm.nih.gov/pmc/articles/PMC3241518/

5 https://www.macmillan.org.uk/healthcare-professionals/news-and-resources/blogs/cancer-care-decades-behind

6 https://www.theguardian.com/science/2024/apr/30/healthy-lifestyle-may-offset-genetics-by-60-and-add-five-years-to-life-study-says

7 https://www.kevinmd.com/2020/05/the-medical-education-question-that-needs-to-be-changed.htmlr

8 https://www.fda.gov/media/143704/download

Futureproof Principle #1: Put Out The Inflammation Fire

1 https://news.cancerresearchuk.org/2013/02/01/feeling-the-heat-the-link-between-inflammation-and-cancer/

2 https://news.cancerresearchuk.org/2013/02/01/feeling-the-heat-the-link-between-inflammation-and-cancer/

3 https://www.frontiersin.org/journals/immunology/articles/10.3389/fimmu.2018.00586/full; https://www.ncbi.nlm.nih.gov/pmc/articles/PMC6457053/; https://www.fallbrookmedicalcenter.com/inflammation-is-the-root-cause-of-many-diseases/

4 https://my.clevelandclinic.org/health/symptoms/21660-inflammation; https://www.health.harvard.edu/blog/why-all-the-buzz-about-inflammation-and-just-how-bad-is-it-202203162705

5 https://news.cancerresearchuk.org/2011/11/16/expert-opinion-professor-fran-balkwill/

6 https://news.cancerresearchuk.org/2019/03/28/inflammation-and-cancer-unravelling-a-150-year-old-mystery/

7 https://link.springer.com/article/10.1007/s12016-021-08899-6

8 https://www.nicswell.co.uk/health-news/children-of-the-90s-more-likely-to-be-overweight-or-obese

9 https://researchbriefings.files.parliament.uk/documents/SN03336/SN03336.pdf

10 https://www.ahajournals.org/doi/10.1161/CIRCRESAHA.119.315896

11 https://journals.plos.org/plosone/article?id=10.1371/journal.pone.0132672

12 https://arcr.niaaa.nih.gov/volume/41/1/natural-recovery-liver-and-other-organs-after-chronic-alcohol-use

13 https://www.ncbi.nlm.nih.gov/pmc/articles/PMC8026081/

14 https://ncbi.nlm.nih.gov/pmc/articles/PMC6996528/

15 https://gero.usc.edu/2024/02/20/fasting-mimicking-diet-biological-age

16 https://www.ncbi.nlm.nih.gov/pmc/articles/PMC6984609/

17 https://www.theguardian.com/society/2023/apr/09/british-doctor-pioneers-low-carb-diet-as-cure-for-obesity-and-type-2-diabetes

18 https://www.ncbi.nlm.nih.gov/pmc/articles/PMC8684375/

19 https://www.neurology.org/doi/10.1212/WNL.0000000000207923

20 https://www.aocs.org/stay-informed/inform-magazine/featured-articles/big-fat-controversy-changing-opinions-about-saturated-fats/

21 https://www.ncbi.nlm.nih.gov/pmc/articles/PMC4836695/

22 https://www.ncbi.nlm.nih.gov/pmc/articles/PMC6024687/

23 https://www.ahajournals.org/doi/full/10.1161/CIR.0000000000000743

24 https://www.health.harvard.edu/heart-health/sugar-substitutes-new-cardiovascular-concerns

25 https://www.ncbi.nlm.nih.gov/pmc/articles/PMC5672138/

26 https://www.ncbi.nlm.nih.gov/pmc/articles/PMC9331555/

27 https://foodinsight.org/everything-you-need-to-know-about-acesulfame-potassium/

28 https://www.ncbi.nlm.nih.gov/pmc/articles/PMC6581265/

29 https://www.hopkinsmedicine.org/health/treatment-tests-and-therapies/hyperbaric-oxygen-therapy

Futureproof Principle #2: Get Stronger, Live Longer

1 https://www.visiblebody.com/learn/muscular/muscle-types;

https://medlineplus.gov/ency/imagepages/19841.htm

2 https://www.mdpi.com/1422-0067/23/7/3501

3 https://www.nature.com/articles/s41585-021-00476-y

4 https://www.cnet.com/health/fitness/how-weightlifting-burns-body-fat-even-after-your-workout/

5 https://medschool.vanderbilt.edu/mstp/2017/05/18/nobel-laureate-eric-kandel-md-gives-vanderbilt-flexner-discovery-lecture/

6 https://www.cdc.gov/injury/features/older-adult-falls/index.html

7 https://ukhsa.blog.gov.uk/2014/07/17/the-human-cost-of-falls/

8 https://ukhsa.blog.gov.uk/2014/07/17/the-human-cost-of-falls/

9 https://ukhsa.blog.gov.uk/2014/07/17/the-human-cost-of-falls/

10 https://www.ageuk.org.uk/latest-press/articles/2019/may/falls-in-later-life-a-huge-concern-for-older-people/

11 https://www.sciencedaily.com/releases/2013/09/130927092350.htm

12 https://www.fitnessgenes.com/blog/your-muscle-hypertrophy-mtor-trait

13 https://onlinelibrary.wiley.com/doi/full/10.1111/cen.13932

14 https://kidshealth.org/en/teens/contraception-depo.html

15 https://www.health.harvard.edu/staying-healthy/strength-training-builds-more-than-muscles

16 https://www.health.harvard.edu/staying-healthy/strength-training-builds-more-than-muscles

17 https://biodensity.com/about

18 https://pmc.ncbi.nlm.nih.gov/articles/PMC4625777/

19 https://www.cityam.com/gogglebox-nation-how-many-hours-do-brits-spend-watching-tv/

20 https://www.freeletics.com/en/blog/posts/3-dimensional-training/

21 https://www.onepeloton.com/blog/ankle-strengthening-exercises/

22 https://www.treadmillreviews.net/benefits-of-decline-training-on-treadmills/#:~:text=Whereas%20incline%20training%20forces%20runners,when%20leaning%20forward%20for%20sprints.

23 https://rucking.com/does-rucking-build-muscle/

24 https://www.ncbi.nlm.nih.gov/pmc/articles/PMC6104107/

25 https://www.graduate.umaryland.edu/gsa/gazette/February-2016/How-the-human-body-uses-electricity/

26 https://www.ncbi.nlm.nih.gov/pmc/articles/PMC2874510/

27 https://nutrigardens.com/blogs/blog/tart-cherry-juice-for-muscle-

recovery-what-you-need-to-know

28 https://www.elo.health/articles/the-best-muscle-recovery-supplements/

29 https://www.healthline.com/nutrition/what-is-creatine#muscle-gain

30 https://barbend.com/salt-pre-workout/

31 https://www.ncbi.nlm.nih.gov/pmc/articles/PMC6778477/

32 https://www.ncbi.nlm.nih.gov/pmc/articles/PMC5789890/

Futureproof Principle #3: Eat For Vitality

1 https://medlineplus.gov/ency/article/002222.htm

2 https://www.hsph.harvard.edu/nutritionsource/collagen/

3 https://www.ncbi.nlm.nih.gov/pmc/articles/PMC6566836/

4 https://www.ncbi.nlm.nih.gov/pmc/articles/PMC6566836/

5 https://www.ncbi.nlm.nih.gov/pmc/articles/PMC6179508/

6 https://assets.publishing.service.gov.uk/media/5bbb790de5274a2241 5d7fee/Eatwell_guide_colour_edition.pdf

7 https://bjsm.bmj.com/content/51/24/1730

8 https://bjsm.bmj.com/content/51/24/1730

9 https://www.zoeharcombe.com/2016/03/eatwell-guide-conflicts-of-interest/

10 https://www.healthline.com/nutrition/22-high-fiber-foods#types-of-fiber

11 https://eu.usatoday.com/story/entertainment/celebrities/2020/04/13/liam-hemsworth-kidney-stone-surgery-mens-health/2981717001/

12 https://news.medill.northwestern.edu/chicago/kale-sheds-bum-rap-on-kidney-stones/; https://www.healthline.com/nutrition/oxalate-good-or-bad

13 https://www.dailymail.co.uk/sciencetech/article-2354580/Popeyes-legendary-love-spinach-actually-misplaced-decimal-point.html

14 https://kidneystones.uchicago.edu/2015/11/16/how-to-eat-a-low-oxalate-diet/

15 https://www.marekdoyle.com/does-magnesium-supplementation-reduce-oxalate-absorption-soluble-vs-insoluble-and-partially-soluble-oxalate-salts-and-why-it-matters/

16 https://www.ohmgwater.com/pages/frequently-asked-questions

17 https://www.npr.org/sections/health-shots/2024/02/18/1231552773/protein-diet-muscle-strength-training-muscle-loss-women

18 https://www.nutritionix.com/food/roasted-chicken-thigh

19 https://www.forbes.com/health/nutrition/high-protein-foods/

20 https://www.healthline.com/nutrition/6-health-benefits-of-hemp-seeds

21 https://microbiomejournal.biomedcentral.com/articles/10.1186/s40168-017-0370-7

22 https://scientificinquirer.com/2022/03/09/food-expeditions-the-maasai-contradiction-healthy-living-on-a-roast-meat-diet/

23 https://www.tesco.com/groceries/en-GB/products/306810938

24 https://sciencedirect.com/science/article/abs/pii/S1568163721002476

25 https://www.verywellhealth.com/collagen-supplements-4164818

26 https://www.healthline.com/nutrition/glycine#TOC_TITLE_HDR_2

27 https://www.ncbi.nlm.nih.gov/pmc/articles/PMC1464262/

28 https://fortune.com/europe/2024/05/01/novo-nordisk-market-value-570-billion-bigger-than-danish-denmark-economy/

29 https://pubmed.ncbi.nlm.nih.gov/32429999/

30 https://integrative-medicine.ca/is-histamine-intolerance-the-culprit-behind-your-skin-condition/

31 https://www.healthline.com/health/beauty-skin-care/collagen-food-boost

32 https://www.ncbi.nlm.nih.gov/pmc/articles/PMC9655929/

33 https://www.ncbi.nlm.nih.gov/pmc/articles/PMC8791758/

34 https://webdoc.agsci.colostate.edu/cepep/FactSheets/201Household Pesticides.pdf

35 https://www.thalgo.com.au/blogs/news/what-is-silicium

36 https://www.ncbi.nlm.nih.gov/pmc/articles/PMC6561714/

37 https://www.ncbi.nlm.nih.gov/pmc/articles/PMC5579659/

38 https://pubmed.ncbi.nlm.nih.gov/28751807/

Futureproof Principle #4: Get Moving

1 https://www.ncbi.nlm.nih.gov/pmc/articles/PMC2996155/

2 https://www.betterhealth.vic.gov.au/health/healthyliving/the-dangers-of-sitting

3 https://www.ncbi.nlm.nih.gov/pmc/articles/PMC2996155/

4 https://www.ncbi.nlm.nih.gov/pmc/articles/PMC6025535/

5 https://www.ncbi.nlm.nih.gov/pmc/articles/PMC2996155/

6 https://www.betterhealth.vic.gov.au/health/healthyliving/the-dangers-

of-sitting

7 https://www.mdanderson.org/publications/focused-on-health/cancer-risk-sitting.h11-1589046.html

8 https://www.nhs.uk/live-well/exercise/why-sitting-too-much-is-bad-for-us/

9 https://www.betterhealth.vic.gov.au/health/healthyliving/the-dangers-of-sitting

10 https://pubmed.ncbi.nlm.nih.gov/27358494/

11 https://pubmed.ncbi.nlm.nih.gov/21846575/

12 https://www.ncbi.nlm.nih.gov/pmc/articles/PMC8765450/

13 https://www.ncbi.nlm.nih.gov/pmc/articles/PMC8230594/

14 https://pubmed.ncbi.nlm.nih.gov/12124860/

15 https://www.nhsfife.org/media/o514vhmp/nhs-fife-toilet-positioning.pdf

16 From *Built to Move*, by Kelly and Juliet Starrett (Orion Spring, 2023).

17 https://www.ncbi.nlm.nih.gov/pmc/articles/PMC6025535/

18 https://www.onnit.com/academy/3-tests-that-prove-why-you-need-to-prioritize-mobility-training/

19 https://www.onnit.com/academy/hack-your-mobility-training-with-these-3-tips/

20 https://www.theguardian.com/lifeandstyle/2024/feb/05/touch-your-toes-six-fast-easy-ways-to-improve-your-mobility-and-live-a-longer-life

21 https://academic.oup.com/eurjpc/article/21/7/892/5925784

22 https://www.health.com/floor-sitting-posture-benefits-7377628

23 https://www.bbc.com/future/article/20230814-why-fidgeting-is-good-for-you

24 https://suffolkandnortheastessex.icb.nhs.uk/news/how-long-can-you-stand-like-a-flamingo/

25 https://diabetesjournals.org/care/article/35/5/976/38374/Breaking-Up-Prolonged-Sitting-Reduces-Postprandial

26 https://www.healthline.com/health-news/science-says-toilet-footstools-really-can-improve-the-way-you-poop

27 https://www.inverse.com/mind-body/grab-a-rope-seven-reasons-why-skipping-is-so-good-for-you

28 https://cks.nice.org.uk/topics/chronic-pain/background-information/prevalence/

29 https://www.statista.com/statistics/521802/otc-pain-relief-treatments-

sales-value-great-britain/

30 https://www.britishpainsociety.org/media-resources/

31 https://my.clevelandclinic.org/health/body/23251-fascia

32 https://my.clevelandclinic.org/health/body/23251-fascia

33 https://pubmed.ncbi.nlm.nih.gov/30252294/

34 https://www.healthline.com/health/fascia-blasting

35 https://birthfit.com/blog/fascia-basics

36 https://www.hopkinsmedicine.org/health/wellness-and-prevention/muscle-pain-it-may-actually-be-your-fascia

37 https://www.healthline.com/health/fascia-blasting

38 https://www.sciencedirect.com/science/article/abs/pii/S1360859209000941

Futureproof Principle #5: Calm The F--- Down

1 https://www.mentalhealth.org.uk/about-us/news/survey-stressed-nation-UK-overwhelmed-unable-to-cope

2 https://sapienlabs.org/wp-content/uploads/2024/03/4th-Annual-Mental-State-of-the-World-Report.pdf

3 https://www.theguardian.com/society/2024/jan/22/mental-health-uk-burnt-out-nation

4 https://mhfaengland.org/mhfa-centre/blog/ten-workplace-mental-health-statistics-for-2023/

5 https://www.britannica.com/science/amygdala

6 https://www.health.harvard.edu/staying-healthy/understanding-the-stress-response

7 https://my.clevelandclinic.org/health/articles/22187-cortisol

8 https://my.clevelandclinic.org/health/articles/22187-cortisol

9 https://www.cell.com/iscience/fulltext/S2589-0042(22)00965-8

10 https://my.clevelandclinic.org/health/body/hypothalamic-pituitary-adrenal-hpa-axis; https://www.liebertpub.com/doi/full/10.1089/ars.2021.0153

11 https://www.health.harvard.edu/staying-healthy/why-stress-causes-people-to-overeat

12 https://www.ncbi.nlm.nih.gov/pmc/articles/PMC371414/

13 https://www.sciencedirect.com/science/article/abs/pii/S2212962614000054

14 https://www.scientificamerican.com/article/how-parents-rsquo-

trauma-leaves-biological-traces-in-children/

15 https://pubmed.ncbi.nlm.nih.gov/18037011/

16 https://www.ncbi.nlm.nih.gov/pmc/articles/PMC3428505/

17 https://pubmed.ncbi.nlm.nih.gov/37086720/

18 https://www.sciencedirect.com/science/article/pii/S0889159122001477

19 https://www.priorygroup.com/mental-health/stress-treatment/stress-statistics

20 https://www.annualreviews.org/content/journals/10.1146/annurev-neuro-091619-022657

21 https://www.sciencedirect.com/science/article/pii/S0149763418308613

22 https://www.runnersworld.com/uk/health/mental-health/a60125903/cortisol-and-exercise/

23 https://www.sciencedirect.com/science/article/abs/pii/S2212962614000054

24 https://www.ncbi.nlm.nih.gov/pmc/articles/PMC9415189/

25 https://www.youtube.com/watch?v=kSZKIupBUuc

26 https://www.bustle.com/wellness/double-inhale-breathing

27 https://www.verywellmind.com/ways-crying-can-improve-your-mental-health-6745650

28 https://www.ncbi.nlm.nih.gov/pmc/articles/PMC6751071/

29 https://www.theguardian.com/society/article/2024/may/13/health-expert-tim-spector-criticised-for-remarks-on-year-round-use-of-sunscreen

31 https://www.instagram.com/p/C5gB0LLOcUM/?igsh=aDU2bXhwNmF4aHo%3D

31 https://www.ncbi.nlm.nih.gov/pmc/articles/PMC2562900/

32 https://www.healthline.com/health/depression/benefits-sunlight

33 https://www.mdpi.com/2072-6643/15/11/2433

34 https://www.verywellhealth.com/red-light-therapy-5217767

35 https://www.verywellhealth.com/red-light-therapy-5217767

36 https://www.ncbi.nlm.nih.gov/pmc/articles/PMC2796659/

37 https://pubmed.ncbi.nlm.nih.gov/29351426/; https://www.bbc.co.uk/programmes/articles/4Q1s9Tyb9ZZmyqZhQk489FS/why-we-should-all-be-taking-cold-showers

38 https://www.businessinsider.com/stress-relief-cold-heat-hiit-short-bursts-help-recovery-2022-3

39 https://www.clearlightsaunas.eu/blog/sauna-liver

40 https://ccare.stanford.edu/uncategorized/connectedness-health-the-science-of-social-connection-infographic/; https://www.health.harvard.edu/staying-healthy/understanding-the-stress-response

41 https://english.elpais.com/science-tech/2023-06-21/a-review-of-studies-with-22-million-people-shows-that-loneliness-increases-the-risk-of-dying.html#

42 https://www.thetimes.co.uk/article/stress-beat-burnout-mo-gawdat-alice-law-unstressable-pl35v2cmn

Futureproof Living: Putting it into action

1 https://www.healthline.com/nutrition/berberine-powerful-supplement#other-benefits

2 https://www.webmd.com/diet/black-seed-health-benefits

3 https://www.ncbi.nlm.nih.gov/pmc/articles/PMC5664031

4 https://www.ncbi.nlm.nih.gov/pmc/articles/PMC7143620/

5 https://www.ncbi.nlm.nih.gov/pmc/articles/PMC4378297/

Conclusion

1 https://www.forbes.com/sites/johnkoetsier/2021/11/02/self-driving-farm-robot-uses-lasers-to-kill-100000-weeds-an-hour-saving-land-and-farmers-from-toxic-herbicides/

2 https://www.instagram.com/dr.joezundell

3 https://www.maramaathome.com/

ABOUT THE AUTHOR

Entrepreneur, biohacking pioneer, weight loss expert and mother of four, Davinia Taylor's career started on television. She turned her life around from being a notorious 90s party girl, biohacking her way to optimum health, losing nearly three stone, and dedicating herself to researching the effect of lifestyle hacks on our bodies. Her food supplement business, WillPowders, helps an ever-confused population crush cravings and achieve genuine wellbeing. Davinia shares her discoveries and learnings through public events and on her rapidly growing Instagram accounts @daviniataylor and @willpowders.